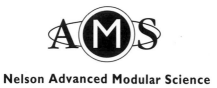

Nelson Advanced Modular Science

Food and Health

JOHN ADDS • ERICA LARKCOM • RUTH MILLER

Nelson

Thomas Nelson & Sons Ltd
Nelson House
Mayfield Road
Walton-on-Thames
Surrey KT12 5PL
United Kingdom

I(T)P   Thomas Nelson is an International Thomson Company
I(T)P   is used under licence

First Published by Thomas Nelson & Sons Ltd 1998
ISBN   0 17 448272 8
9 8 7 6 5 4 3 2 1
01 00 99 98

Typesetting and illustration by Hardlines, Charlbury, Oxfordshire
Printed by Eurografica S.p.A., Vicenza, Italy
Picture Research by Image Select International Ltd

Publication team:
Acquisitions: Sonia Clark
Editorial management: Simon Bell
Freelance editorial: Liz Jones
Production: Suzanne Howarth
Marketing: Jane Lewis

Acknowledgements

The authors and publishers would like to thank the following for permission to
reproduce copyright images.
Erica Larkcom: figures 3.1, 3.4, 3.13, 3.16, 4.1, 4.9, 4.12a, b and c, 4.13a and b, 4.17a, b and c
Tropix Photo Library: figure 1.6 (M. & V. Birley); figure 1.8 (P. Frances);
Science Photo Library: figure 1.7 (Peter Menzel);
Chris Fairclough Colour Library/Image Select: figure 2.7;
Tony Stone Images: figure 3.9 (Duncan Wherrett)
National Dairy Council: figure 4.7 a, b and c (Gary Bellamy)
John Innes Centre: 4.18a
IACR - Long Ashton Research Station: figure 4.18b
The authors and publishers would also like to thank the following for their help in the
preparation of this book:
John Schollar, Dean Madden, The National Centre for Biotechnology Education,
The British Nutrition Foundation, Sainsburys plc
The examination questions and mark schemes on pages 92–97 appear by permission
of Edexcel (London Examinations)

Contents

Introduction

As modularisation of syllabuses gains momentum, there is a corresponding demand for a modular format in supporting texts. The Nelson Advanced Modular Science series has been written by Chief and Principal Examiners and those involved directly with the A level examinations. The books are based on the London Examinations (Edexcel) AS and A level modular syllabuses in Biology and Human Biology, Chemistry and Physics. Each module text offers complete and self-contained coverage of all the topics in the module. The texts also include examples outside the prescribed syllabus to broaden your understanding and help to illustrate the principle which is being presented. There are practical investigations and regular review questions to stimulate your thinking while you read about and study the topic. Finally, there are typical examination questions with mark schemes so that you can test yourself and help you to understand how to approach the examination.

In the Option modules of the London syllabuses, we explore applications of Biology, delving into some areas where we really make use of biology in our everyday lives. In Food and Health, the focus is on the origins of food as biological material, and the effects of the human diet on health. We look first at food inside the human body, considering the nature of different components of the diet and the biological effects of both under nutrition and overnutrition. Links between diet and certain health disorders are illustrated by coronary heart disease, diseases of the colon and diabetes mellitus. Special reference is made to the effects on health of additives and of sugars in the diet. The second theme in the book follows the events which occur in typical raw foods from the time of harvest through to their presentation to the consumer on the supermarket shelf or market stall. An understanding of the biological changes after harvest in fruit, vegetables and meat is developed in the context of delaying deterioration and avoiding microbial spoilage in food materials. We see how storage systems are manipulated to prolong the shelf life of fresh foods. We then look closely at packaging as a means of containing, protecting and controlling the postharvest changes in food materials. The contribution to the food industry of biotechnology (ancient and modern) is reviewed through a range of fermentations - sauerkraut, soya sauce, yoghurt and cheese, bread and wine - with a glimpse into the future potential for using gene technology in food production. The authors hope that through your study of topics in this book, you will develop an understanding of the biology of changes which occur naturally in raw fresh foods before they get channelled into the food processing industry, and are able to make informed decisions about the relationships between different human diets and health.

The authors

Erica Larkcom B.A., M.A., C.Biol., M.I.Biol., Subject Officer for A level Biology, formerly Head of Biology, Great Cornard Upper School, Suffolk

John Adds B.A., C.Biol., M.I.Biol., Dip. Ed., Chief Examiner for A level Biology, Head of Biology, Abbey Tutorial College, London

Ruth Miller B.Sc., C.Biol., M.I.Biol., Chief Examiner for AS and A level Biology, formerly Head of Biology, Sir William Perkins's School, Chertsey, Surrey

Note to teachers on safety

When practical instructions have been given we have attempted to indicate hazardous substances and operations by using standard symbols and appropriate precautions. Nevertheless you should be aware of your obligations under the Health and Safety at Work Act, Control of Substances Hazardous to Health (COSHH) Regulations and the Management of Health and Safety at Work Regulations. In this respect you should follow the requirements of your employers at all times.

In carrying out practical work, students should be encouraged to carry out their own risk assessments, i.e. they should identify hazards and suitable ways of reducing the risks from them. However, they must be checked by the teacher/lecturer. Students must also know what to do in an emergency, such as a fire.

The teachers/lecturers should be familiar and up to date with current advice from professional bodies.

Food and diet

Human beings, in common with other **heterotrophic** organisms, require a supply of ready-made organic compounds in order to obtain sufficient energy and materials to sustain life. **Autotrophic** organisms, on the other hand, synthesise the organic compounds they require from simple, inorganic molecules, in processes which use either light or chemical energy. Algae, green plants and some prokaryotes are able to build up carbohydrates, lipids and proteins from carbon dioxide, mineral ions and water, using energy from the sun in a process called **photosynthesis**. The light energy is absorbed by special pigments and converted into chemical energy. In green plants, the pigments are chlorophylls, present in chloroplasts in the cells of the leaves. Details of the process of photosynthesis can be found in *The Organism and the Environment*.

Because of their ability to use energy from the sun in the synthesis of organic compounds, photosynthetic organisms are known as **primary producers**. All heterotrophic organisms are **consumers** and depend, directly or indirectly, on the producers for their supplies of organic compounds. Plant-eaters, the **herbivores**, are **primary consumers** and obtain all their nutrients from green plants. **Secondary consumers** are **carnivores** and feed on the primary consumers. Heterotrophic organisms that obtain their food from both plant and animal sources are known as omnivores. Most human beings are **omnivores**, feeding on a mixture of products from plant and animal sources. The consumption of meat and meat products by human beings varies and is often affected by social and religious factors. Many groups, including Muslims and Jews, never eat pork or products from pigs; Hindus and Sikhs do not eat beef. **Vegetarians** eat no meat, but many include milk, milk products and eggs in their diets. **Vegans**, who only eat food from plant sources and consume no animal products at all, can be considered as herbivores.

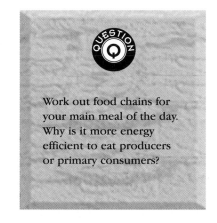

Work out food chains for your main meal of the day. Why is it more energy efficient to eat producers or primary consumers?

If we, as consumers, look closely at the origins of the food we eat, we can trace it back to a plant source in a sequence known as a **food chain**. Each organism in the chain occupies a particular trophic level. Most of these food chains are fairly short, consisting of two or three **trophic levels**, as most of our food is derived directly from plants or from animals that eat plants. More examples of food chains and information about the interrelationships between autotrophic and heterotrophic organisms can be found in *The Organism and the Environment*.

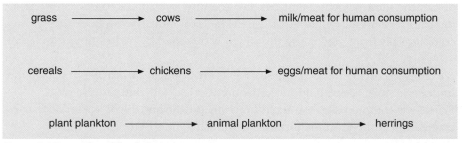

grass ⟶ cows ⟶ milk/meat for human consumption

cereals ⟶ chickens ⟶ eggs/meat for human consumption

plant plankton ⟶ animal plankton ⟶ herrings

Figure 1.1 Examples of food chains

Nutritional requirements

A healthy human diet should provide:
- sufficient energy-providing foods to enable the body to carry out internal processes and external activities
- sufficient materials for growth and for the repair and replacement of cells and tissues.

In addition, some of the nutrients we obtain from our food provide substances that are needed to maintain the internal processes of the body.
These dietary requirements are met by the inclusion of five types of nutrients:
- carbohydrates
- lipids (fats)
- proteins
- mineral ions
- vitamins

together with water and dietary fibre (NSP).

For the details of the chemical nature of these nutrients, reference should be made to the relevant chapter in *Cell Biology and Genetics*. In this chapter, the emphasis is on the functions of these nutrients in the body and their sources in our food.

Carbohydrates

Carbohydrates are one of the major groups of nutrients in the human diet. The **monosaccharide** glucose is the main respiratory substrate in the body and a constant supply is required to maintain the metabolic activities of the cells and tissues. Most of the carbohydrate in our diet is in the form of **disaccharides**, such as sucrose and lactose, or **polysaccharides**, such as starch and cellulose, although some monosaccharides are present in fruits. The disaccharides and starch are digested, yielding monosaccharides which are absorbed from the small intestine into the blood, but we do not produce enzymes which are able to digest cellulose. Some of the cellulose in the fibre in our diet may be broken down by bacteria present in the colon.

Glucose occurs naturally in grapes and other sweet fruits, onions, tomatoes and honey. **Fructose** also occurs in honey and sweet fruit juices. Monosaccharides do not have to be digested and can be absorbed into the blood from the small intestine. Both glucose and fructose are sweet-tasting, but compared with sucrose, glucose tastes less sweet and fructose tastes twice as sweet. Using fructose instead of sucrose in food products, it is possible to obtain the same sweetness for half the quantity, so manufacturers can reduce the calorie content. Fructose for use in the food industry can be made commercially from glucose syrup, which is obtained by hydrolysing starch.

Naturally occurring disaccharides, such as **sucrose** and **maltose** in plants and **lactose** in milk, are also important sources of carbohydrate in the diet. Sucrose is commercially extracted from sugar cane and sugar beet, and is used extensively in the food manufacturing industry. Sucrose is also present in a large number of fruits, grasses and roots. Maltose occurs naturally in

What do you think is meant by the term 'hidden sugars'? How many of the goods you consume contain such sugars? You should check the labels.

germinating seeds. It is extracted from germinating barley grains and used in the manufacture of beer. The lactose in milk provides young mammals with about 40 per cent of their energy requirements. Cow's milk contains about 5 per cent lactose and human milk about 8 per cent. Some people, said to be **lactose intolerant**, are unable to produce enough of the enzyme lactase, which digests lactose. Undigested lactose passes into the large intestine, where it is converted into lactic acid by bacteria, causing diarrhoea. This condition can occur in babies and small children, but it is widespread in the adult populations of Asia, Africa and Eastern Europe, where about three-quarters of the adult population develop it between the ages of 15 and 25. In Western Europe, milk has traditionally been part of the adult diet and most people retain the ability to produce lactase throughout their lives, but in other parts of the world milk is only given to babies and young children. Milk products, such as cheese and yoghurt, contain little lactose and can be digested without causing discomfort.

Disaccharides in the diet are digested by enzymes in the walls of the duodenum and the ileum. The products are monosaccharides, which are absorbed into the blood. The enzymes and the products of digestion are shown in Table 1.1.

Oligosaccharides are polysaccharides made up of three to ten monosaccharide units and are present in cereal grains and in vegetables, such as peas, beans, leeks, onions and garlic. These compounds pass through the gut to the large intestine, as we do not produce the enzymes necessary for their digestion. Some bacteria, particularly *Bifidobacteria* and *Lactobacillus*, present in the large intestine, are able to break down the oligosaccharides, producing short-chain fatty acids, carbon dioxide and hydrogen. The presence of the oligosaccharides in the diet promotes the growth of these beneficial bacteria at the expense of harmful bacteria, such as *Clostridium* and the coliform bacteria, which are responsible for infections in the gut.

The polysaccharide **starch** is the main carbohydrate storage compound in plants. It can be found in a variety of plant parts, including stems, roots and tubers. It is particularly abundant in the parenchyma tissue of stem tubers of the potato (*Solanum tuberosum*), the endosperm of cereal grains and the cotyledons of seeds of the Papilionaceae (legumes). The starch is found in the form of grains or granules, within cells and these grains can vary in size and shape within a tissue.

Most of the starchy food we eat is cooked. Uncooked starch is very difficult to digest, because the starch grains are contained within the cellulose cell walls of the plant tissue and thus inaccessible to our digestive enzymes. Once the tissue is cooked, the cell walls are softened, allowing water to penetrate and act on the starch grains and causing them to begin to break down and gelatinise. This starch can then be digested by amylase, either in the saliva or in the pancreatic juice. The starch is broken down to maltose, which is further digested to glucose by maltase in the walls of the ileum.

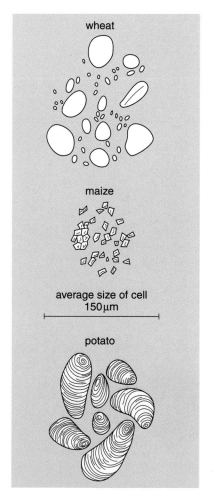

Figure 1.2 Different types of starch grains in cells

FOOD AND DIET

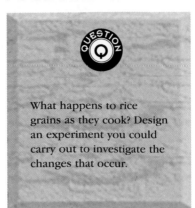

What happens to rice grains as they cook? Design an experiment you could carry out to investigate the changes that occur.

Table 1.1 *The digestion of some carbohydrates in the diet*

Carbohydrate	Digestive enzymes and location of digestion	Products of digestion
sucrose (disaccharide)	sucrase in walls of small intestine	glucose and fructose
maltose (disaccharide)	maltase in walls of small intestine	glucose
lactose (disaccharide)	lactase in walls of small intestine	glucose and galactose
starch (polysaccharide)	salivary amylase in mouth, pancreatic amylase in duodenum	maltose (which is digested by maltase in the small intestine)

The **digestibility** of the starch in our diets varies according to its source and treatment. The most rapidly digested starch is found in bread, some breakfast cereals and freshly-cooked potatoes. The cereal grains, which are used in the manufacture of some breakfast cereals and in flour used for baking, are subjected to **milling**, which breaks open the cell walls, releasing the starch granules. In addition, these foods have usually been cooked, so the starch is more easily digested by the amylase present in the duodenum and the ileum. The starch present in whole grain cereals, beans, peas, lentils and pasta takes longer to be digested because the granules are still contained within the cells or, in the case of pasta, the product has a very dense structure. Some of the starch in these foods, referred to as **resistant starch**, is not digested by the amylase and passes through the small intestine to the colon, where it is used by the bacteria there in much the same way as the oligosaccharides. This is starch that is either still contained within plant cells (peas, lentils, sweetcorn, whole cereal grains) or present in a crystalline form resistant to digestion (bananas). The starch in foods that have been processed by cooking and then allowed to cool, may also become transformed into a resistant starch.

Non-starch polysaccharides (NSPs) are carbohydrates which come from the cell walls of plants. They include **cellulose**, which is insoluble in water, together with water-soluble pectins, hemi-celluloses and gums. These substances were previously referred to as 'roughage' or 'dietary fibre', although neither term accurately describes their nature nor the role they play in the diet. Dietary fibre used to be defined as 'material derived from plant cell walls in foods', but this was later modified to 'the skeletal remnants of plant cell walls resistant to digestion by the enzymes of humans'. Foods which are high in NSP are usually derived from cereal grains. Wheat, maize and rice yield mostly cellulose, which is insoluble, but oats, barley and rye contain a higher proportion of soluble NSP. We also obtain non-starch polysaccharides from the fruit and vegetables we eat, but the water content is higher, making the NSP content lower. Table 1.2. shows the NSP of some natural and processed foods.

It is relevant to note the difference in NSP of white and wholemeal bread, where the use of the whole grains increases the NSP five-fold.

Table 1.2 *The non-starch polysaccharide content of some natural and processed foods (The NSP is measured in g per 100 g of food)*

Food	Soluble NSP	Insoluble NSP	Total NSP
apples	0.72	1.21	1.93
potatoes	0.54	0.5	1.04
carrots	0.92	1.02	1.94
baked beans	1.70	1.50	3.20
white bread	1.16	0.44	1.60
wholemeal bread	1.66	4.55	6.21
rolled oats	3.58	2.91	6.49
corn flakes	0.17	0.47	0.64
Kellogg's All Bran	3.74	18.73	22.47

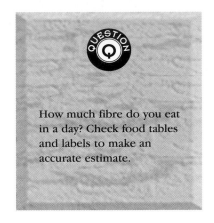

How much fibre do you eat in a day? Check food tables and labels to make an accurate estimate.

The inclusion of significant amounts of NSP in the diet does have beneficial effects on health. For a long time, it has been known that NSP speeds up the passage of food through the gut ('transit time'), thus promoting regular bowel movements. The stools are larger and softer, possibly due to the absorption of water by the NSP, and so easier to pass. On a typical British diet, the transit time is usually about 100 hours, but this can be reduced to 36 hours if the diet is high in NSP. There is a considerable body of evidence to show that a diet high in NSP can help prevent many bowel diseases such as constipation, diverticular disease, cancer of the colon and haemorrhoids, because of the speeding up of the transit time. High quantities of soluble NSP may help reduce the blood cholesterol level in certain people and this may contribute to lowering the incidence of coronary heart disease.

The NSP found in cereal grains is associated with compounds which form complexes with mineral ions. The uptake and absorption of mineral ions from the small intestine is not as efficient and so people whose diet is high in NSP and low in minerals could show signs of mineral deficiency. It is recommended that a healthy diet should contain at least 18 g of NSP per day for adults and that this should come from a range of foods such as fruit, vegetables and cereals, so that it includes both soluble and insoluble NSP. An upper limit of 32 g of NSP per day is recommended, to avoid the drawback associated with too much fibre.

NSP is not digested by the digestive enzymes present in the alimentary canal, so it passes unchanged through the stomach and small intestine. When it reaches the large intestine, it is used by the bacteria there, resulting in the formation of short chain fatty acids, carbon dioxide, hydrogen and methane. Some of the short chain fatty acids are absorbed and can be metabolised by the body.

Lipids

The term 'lipid' is used to describe a group of naturally occurring fat-like compounds, which are insoluble in water but soluble in organic solvents such as alcohol and ether. **Oils** and **fats** are **triglycerides (triacylglycerols)**, formed from the condensation of glycerol and three fatty acid molecules.

There is no difference in the composition of oils and fats, but they are distinguished by their state at normal room temperature: usually fats are solid and oils are liquid. They form the major stores and sources of energy, having a higher available energy content (37 kJ g^{-1}) than either carbohydrates or proteins (17 kJ g^{-1}). They provide the fat-soluble vitamins A, D, E and K and, on digestion, they provide the body with **essential fatty acids (EFA's)**. EFA's are needed for synthesis and cannot be provided from other constituents of the diet. Only small amounts are needed (2 to 4 g per day) so deficiencies are unlikely to occur in normal individuals eating a balanced diet. Fat acts as a carrier of flavour and aromatic compounds and so its presence makes food more palatable.

Phospholipids have a different structure from fats. Only two of the hydroxyl groups of the glycerol are combined with fatty acids, the third is combined with a complex containing a phosphate group. Phospholipids are concerned with the transport of lipids in the blood and are also important constituents of cell membranes.

Cholesterol is a fat-like substance present in animal tissues. We do obtain a certain amount from the food we eat, but we also make it, especially in the liver. It is present in all cell membranes and is also needed for the synthesis of bile acids and some hormones.

It is of relevance here to consider the different types of fatty acids which may be present in the triglycerides which form part of our diet. There are three types, **saturated, mono-unsaturated (MUFA)** and **polyunsaturated (PUFA)**, differing in structure due to the number of double bonds in the carbon chain. The differences and examples are given in Table 1.3.

Table 1.3 *The differences in structure between saturated and unsaturated fatty acids*

Type of fatty acid	Number of double bonds in the carbon chain	Example
saturated	none	stearic acid $CH_3(CH_2)_{16}COOH$
mono-unsaturated (MUFA)	one $-CH=CH-$	oleic acid $CH_3(CH_2)_7CH=CH(CH_2)_7COOH$
polyunsaturated (PUFA)	two or more $-CH=CH-CH_2-CH=CH-$	linoleic acid $CH_3(CH_2)_4CH=CHCH_2CH=CH(CH_2)_7COOH$

All naturally occurring fats contain both saturated and unsaturated fatty acids. Fats such as butter, which have a higher proportion of saturated fatty acids, are solid at room temperature, whereas those which have a higher proportion of unsaturated fatty acids, such as olive oil, are liquid at room temperature. The more double bonds present in the carbon chains of the constituent fatty acid molecules, the lower the melting point of the fat. Fats obtained from animal sources usually contain a higher proportion of saturated fatty acids than the vegetable oils, although it should be noted that fish oils are very high in PUFAs. Palm oil and coconut oil are high in saturated fatty acids.

In order to function efficiently, the body needs certain fatty acids which it cannot synthesise. These are known as **essential fatty acids**. They are involved with cholesterol metabolism, the synthesis of some hormones and with the structure of cell membranes. These fatty acids are all PUFAs and have to be obtained from the diet. They are present in large quantities in foods such as vegetable oils, nuts and soft margarine, and it is very rare for there to be a deficiency in a normal person's diet.

Unsaturated fatty acids exist in two forms: the *cis* form, where the two parts of the hydrocarbon chain are on the same side of the double bond, and the *trans* form, where the two parts are on opposite sides of the double bond. Those naturally occurring unsaturated fatty acids which are essential fatty acids, have the *cis* form, but the corresponding *trans* forms are unable to act as essential fatty acids as they are not recognised by enzymes in the body. The significance in our diet is that the process of hydrogenation of oils, used in the manufacture of margarine, brings about the conversion of some of the unsaturated fatty acids to saturated fatty acids and also converts the naturally occurring *cis* forms into *trans* forms. Similar changes can be brought about by heating. The body deals with these *trans* forms of unsaturated fatty acids in the same way as the saturated fatty acids.

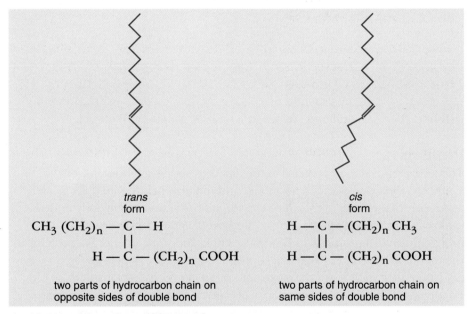

Fig 1.3 Cis and trans forms of fatty acids

The digestion of fats occurs mostly in the duodenum and the ileum. There is no digestion of fats in the mouth or the stomach, although the heat of the body may convert some solid fat into a liquid state, forming fat globules. In the duodenum, the food is mixed with bile from the liver and pancreatic juice from the pancreas. Bile, which is produced by the liver cells and stored in the gall bladder prior to release, contains salts (especially sodium glycocholate and sodium taurocholate), which lower the surface tension of the fat globules. This has the effect of bringing about emulsification, so that tiny droplets are formed. Lipase, present in the pancreatic juice, hydrolyses fats to their constituent fatty acids and glycerol. Emulsification by bile salts increases the surface area available for the action of lipase, making digestion more efficient.

The absorption of fatty acids and glycerol differs from that of the other products of digestion. As they enter the columnar epithelial cells of the villi, they recombine to form fats which pass into the lacteals. These fats then combine with proteins and other lipids, forming lipoproteins called chylomicrons, which will eventually pass from the lymphatic system into the bloodstream by means of the thoracic lymphatic duct. In the blood plasma, an enzyme hydrolyses these lipoproteins, releasing fatty acids and glycerol, which may be used in respiration or stored as fat in the liver, muscles or in the adipose tissue beneath the skin and around the body organs.

In addition to chylomicrons, there are three other types of lipoproteins found in the blood plasma, all of which are involved in the transport of lipids around the body. They are distinguished from each other by their composition and different densities, which are shown in Table 1.4. Much interest has been shown in the levels of these lipoproteins in the blood and whether they play a role in the risk of developing coronary heart disease.

Table 1.4 *The composition of the lipoproteins present in blood*

Type of lipoprotein	Triglyceride	Phospholipid	Cholesterol	Protein
chylomicron	85	9	4	2
very low density (VLDL)	50	18	22	10
low density (LDL)	10	20	45	25
high density (HDL)	4	24	17	55

Proteins

The primary function of proteins in the diet is to supply amino acids for the synthesis of enzymes, certain hormones and the materials required for growth and repair of the body tissues. Amino acids are not stored in the body in the same way that carbohydrates and fats are stored, and excess amino acids are broken down in a process which produces urea and some energy. So, proteins in the diet have a secondary role as a supplementary source of energy. On oxidation, they yield about the same amount of energy as carbohydrates, 17 kJg^{-1}. For details of the structure of amino acids and of protein synthesis, reference should be made to the relevant sections in *Cell Biology and Genetics*.

The protein in our diet is usually supplied from both plant and animal sources. Plant proteins are obtained from cereal grains, nuts and seeds, whereas animal proteins are present in meat, fish, eggs and dairy products. Plants are able to synthesise all the amino acids they require. Animals obtain amino acids from plants and are also able to synthesise some of their own, by transamination, from those they take in. **Transamination** involves the transfer of the amino group from an amino acid to a Krebs cycle (organic) acid, forming a different amino acid. Mammals, including human beings, are unable to synthesise some amino acids and these must be obtained from the diet. These are termed **essential amino acids** or **indispensable amino acids**.

The **nutritional value** of a protein depends on the variety of its constituent amino acids, together with its biological value (BV) and digestibility. Animal protein, such as is found in meat, eggs and milk, contains all the essential (indispensable) amino acids in the quantities required by an adult, so it is considered to be high-quality protein. In other foods, such as cereals and legumes, one or more of the essential amino acids may be lacking or not present in sufficient quantities. Where this is the case, the amino acid that is at its lowest level is referred to as the **limiting amino acid**. The deficiency of this amino acid will have an effect on the proteins that can be made in the body. For example, methionine is an essential amino acid, which is low in peas and beans. Low levels of methionine in a diet will limit the use of other amino acids, because as the polypeptide chains are built up, once the code for methionine is reached, protein synthesis will stop. Any amino acids coded for after methionine in that polypeptide will not be used. So, low levels, or the absence of one essential amino acid, eventually prevents the use of the others, leading to protein malnutrition. There is usually no problem in obtaining all the essential amino acids as normal diets contain a mixture of protein foods, some of plant and some of animal origin. Foods that lack one of the essential amino acids may be eaten with others that lack a different essential amino acid. A meal containing legumes (lacking methionine) eaten with bread (lacking lysine) or sweetcorn (lacking tryptophan) would supply all the essential amino acids. This is known as the complementary action of proteins.

The **biological value (BV)** of a protein is defined as the percentage of absorbed protein that is retained in the body, available to be converted into body protein. This value can be calculated by measuring the nitrogen intake and then measuring the amounts of nitrogen lost in the urine and in the faeces. The nitrogen lost in the urine represents nitrogen that has been absorbed and used, but not retained, by the body. The nitrogen lost in the faeces has not been absorbed by the body.

So,

$$BV = \frac{\text{nitrogen intake} - (\text{nitrogen lost in urine} + \text{nitrogen lost in faeces})}{\text{nitrogen intake} - \text{nitrogen lost in faeces}} \times 100$$

$$= \frac{\text{nitrogen retained}}{\text{nitrogen absorbed}} \times 100$$

The **net protein utilisation (NPU)** is often used to describe the value of a protein and is defined as the percentage of protein eaten that is retained in the body. It is calculated by measuring the nitrogen intake and nitrogen retained.

$$NPU = \frac{\text{nitrogen retained}}{\text{nitrogen intake}} \times 100$$

This is equivalent to the biological value × digestibility.

Most proteins have a high digestibility and their BV and NPU values are close. Animal proteins, such as those present in eggs, milk, meat and fish, are easily digested but the digestibility of plant protein foods is lower, due to the

pyruvic acid (keto acid) — structure with COOH, C=O, CH$_3$

glutamic acid (amino acid) — structure with COOH, HC—NH$_2$, CH$_2$, CH$_2$, COOH

alanine (amino acid) — structure with COOH, HC—NH$_2$, CH$_3$

α ketoglutaric acid (keto acid) — structure with COOH, C=O, CH$_2$, CH$_2$, COOH

The amino group NH$_2$ is transferred from glutamic acid to pyruvic acid.
Alanine, a different amino acid, is formed.

Fig. 1.4 Transamination

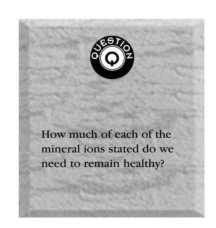

QUESTION

How much of each of the mineral ions stated do we need to remain healthy?

proportion of fibre which tends to increase the removal of nitrogen in the faeces. This is not of significance in a balanced mixed diet, but needs to be considered when the diet does not include animal products.

Mineral ions

Mineral ions are needed in much smaller quantities in the diet than carbohydrates, lipids and proteins. Mineral ions are needed for growth and repair of tissues and are also involved in a range of metabolic processes in the body. Mineral ions such as **calcium** and **phosphate**, are involved in the structure of the bones of the skeleton, **iron** is needed for the formation of haemoglobin in the blood and **sodium** and **chloride** ions are present in blood plasma and other body fluids. Mineral ions are also important as co-factors for enzymes and enzyme activators. Vitamins are also involved in different body processes. The sources of mineral ions and vitamins in our diet, their roles and results of their deficiency in the diet are discussed in the chapter on heterotrophic nutrition (Chapter 2) in *The Organism and the Environment*.

Some mineral ions, such as sodium, potassium and chloride, are present as soluble salts in our food and readily absorbed into the blood from the small intestine. Other necessary ions are not as soluble and tend to form associations with other compounds, making them less available. To illustrate this problem, the absorption of iron and calcium will be considered.

We obtain most of our **iron** from meat, cereals and vegetables, but it is only present in these foods in very small amounts and much of what we ingest passes through the gut without being absorbed. Most adults, eating a diverse diet, only absorb about 15 per cent of the iron present in their food. The amount of absorption is influenced by:
- the source of the iron, whether it is from meat (haem iron) or from plant material (non-haem iron)
- the presence of inhibitors or enhancers of absorption
- the amount of iron already stored in the body.

The iron in meat is organically bound and is absorbed much more readily than the non-haem iron present in plants. This has implications for vegetarians: their dietary intake of iron should be increased to compensate for the lower absorption. Events such as menstruation and pregnancy in women, or a haemorrhage, will increase the absorption of iron. Non-haem iron can combine with other components of the diet, such as phosphates and phytic acid (present in whole cereal grains), resulting in the formation of insoluble salts which cannot be absorbed. However, iron absorption is increased in the presence of vitamin C and alcohol. Vitamin C reduces ferric forms of iron to ferrous forms, which are more easily absorbed. On the other hand, tea causes the formation of insoluble tannic acid salts with iron, inhibiting uptake.

The most important sources of **calcium** and **phosphate** ions are bread, flour, milk and dairy products. The calcium in milk is absorbed readily, due to the presence of lactose which keeps it soluble. Some calcium ions are present in drinking water and significant amounts are consumed in 'hard' water areas, where there are large quantities of calcium sulphate and calcium bicarbonate in the domestic water supplies. A large proportion of the calcium needed by an adult is obtained from processed cereal grains used to make flour and bread. In the process of milling cereal grains, there are significant losses of mineral ions and other nutrients and, in Britain, chalk (calcium carbonate) is added to flour to increase the calcium content, unless the flour is made from whole grains. So white bread is higher in calcium than brown bread. Calcium is absorbed through the lining of the small intestine. The ions bind with a special protein, known as a **calcium-binding protein**, which is present in the intestinal mucosa. The presence of vitamin D is necessary for the formation of the calcium–protein complex: most cases of poor calcium absorption, which may lead to rickets in children or a condition known as osteomalacia in adults, are more often due to a deficiency of vitamin D than shortage of calcium in the diet. In addition, the absorption of calcium can be inhibited by the presence of several factors, including:

- phytic acid, found in whole cereal grains
- oxalates, found in rhubarb and spinach.

These compounds react with the calcium to form insoluble compounds, which cannot be absorbed.

Sodium chloride, or **salt**, is an important component of the diet as it is needed for the normal functioning of the body. The sodium ions help to maintain the volume and osmotic pressure of the blood and of the tissue fluids. In addition, sodium ions are needed for the conduction of nerve impulses and help in the transport of carbon dioxide in the blood. In Britain, the average person takes in about 9 g of salt each day with their food. Excess dietary intake is lost in the urine and in the sweat. There is some evidence to show that a high dietary intake of salt is linked with hypertension (raised blood pressure). This relationship is open to debate, but reducing the salt intake in some hypertensive people has brought about a significant reduction in their blood pressure. We do eat more salt than we need to replace that which is lost each day and it has been recommended that salt intake should be restricted to 6 g per day. Babies need very little salt and will become dehydrated if too much is given in their food. Baby-food manufacturers have made significant reductions in the amount of salt added to their products, as it has been shown that if children develop a taste for salty foods, it is difficult to cut down later in life.

Vitamins

Vitamins are complex organic compounds needed by the body in very small quantities. Most vitamins need to be provided in the diet, although vitamin D can be made in the body by the action of sunlight on the skin and vitamin B6 can be produced from the amino acid tryptophan. Vitamins are more easily absorbed than mineral ions, but the absorption of **nicotinic acid** may be poor where maize forms a large part of the diet. In maize, this vitamin is associated with hemicelluloses in a complex which is not digested by the body, but it can be released by treatment with alkalis. In Mexico, lime-water is used in the preparation of foods containing maize, but in other parts of the world, where there is a high consumption of maize, this is not always done and the population may show signs of the deficiency disease **pellagra**.

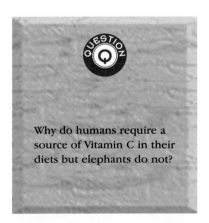

Why do humans require a source of Vitamin C in their diets but elephants do not?

Water

Water may be lost from the body in the following ways:

- as water vapour in exhaled breath from the lungs
- in sweat
- in urine
- in faeces
- in vomit or diarrhoea as a result of illness.

The quantity of water lost from the body will vary according to the climate and the amount of physical exertion. If the climate is hot, then we produce more sweat as a way of controlling the body temperature. Evaporation of the water in sweat cools the surface of the body. Similarly, an increase in manual work or physical exercise will increase heat production in the body and cause the temperature to rise, resulting in more sweat production. Physical exercise also increases the ventilation rate, so more water vapour will be lost from the lungs. Water loss in the urine is variable. If we take in more water than we need, then the excess is removed by the kidneys. If less water is taken in, the urine becomes more concentrated and eventually dehydration could occur. As almost all the processes in the body require water, the consequences of dehydration are serious and the inclusion of fluids in the diet is essential. People can only survive for a few days without water, but will live for about six weeks if deprived of food only. In addition to replacing fluids lost from the body, water can be a source of mineral ions such as calcium and fluorine. In the diet, water comes mainly from the fluids we drink, but a significant quantity is present in our food, particularly in fresh fruit and vegetables.

Balanced diet

A balanced diet is generally understood to be one which provides adequate quantities of all the nutrients required by the body and sufficient energy for optimum growth and health. Lack of a particular nutrient could cause a deficiency disease or lead to malnutrition. In the developed world, deficiency diseases are rare as most people eat a wide variety of foods in sufficient quantities – often in greater quantities than they need so that over-nutrition is common. The quantity of nutrients and energy needed by an individual varies according to their age, gender, body size and level of physical activity.

A diet can be described in terms of its **energy density** and its **nutrient density**. The energy density of a food is determined by the amount of dietary energy provided per unit mass. Foods which provide large amounts of dietary energy have high energy density. If we compare the amount of energy provided by 100 g of chips (1065 kJ) with 100 g of boiled potatoes (343 kJ), we can see that for the same mass of food, the chips provide the larger amount of energy. The chips have a higher energy density than the boiled potatoes.

The nutrient density is determined by the concentrations of useful nutrients in a known mass of food and it is useful to be able to compare different foods on the basis of nutrients supplied per unit of energy. Table 1.5 compares the calcium and energy content of three common foods, white bread, boiled potatoes and milk. It can be seen that the white bread supplies the greatest quantity of energy, but milk supplies the most calcium per 1000 kJ, so it is the most 'calcium' dense.

Is your diet nutrient-dense or energy-dense? Work out a balance sheet of energy intake and energy expenditure.

Table 1.5 *Calcium and energy content of white bread, boiled potatoes and milk*

Food	Energy / kJ per 100 g	Calcium / mg per 1000 kJ
white bread	991	101
boiled potatoes	343	12
milk	272	441

Similar comparisons can be made for all foods. All foods supply some energy and most will supply some nutrients, although it is worth noting that spirits, such as gin and whisky, together with refined white sugar contain no essential nutrients and only supply energy. Other refined or processed foods tend to have a low nutrient density, although their energy density may be high. In a healthy balanced diet, the aim should be to maintain a high nutrient density, so that all the essential nutrients are included, but to keep the energy density low. This usually involves keeping the fat and sugar content of the diet low and including plenty of fruit, vegetables and starchy foods such as bread, rice and pasta. People who use up a lot of energy, due to their occupation or extra physical activity, may need to increase the proportion of energy dense foods in their diets to satisfy their energy needs.

The rate at which the body uses up energy is called the **metabolic rate**. This rate varies throughout the day, according to our activities, and also throughout our lives. A constant supply of energy is used to maintain the essential body processes, such as the pumping of the heart, ventilation, the maintenance of body temperature and chemical processes. These processes go on all the time, even when we are completely at rest. The energy needed for these essential processes is called the basal **metabolic rate (BMR)**, and is determined by our body mass and composition. These factors vary with age and according to gender, with males having higher basal metabolic rates than females. The basal metabolic rate is determined either directly, by measuring heat loss from the body, or indirectly as oxygen consumption per unit time. It is measured when a person is completely at rest in warm conditions and has been fasting for at least 12 hours. As heat energy loss is related to the surface area of the body, basal metabolic rate is expressed as $kJ\ m^{-2}\ h^{-1}$, but it is now considered adequate to define this in terms of the body mass. Thus, BMR can be expressed as kJ of heat energy produced per kg of body mass.

Table 1.6. gives values for the basal metabolic rate in males and females with different body masses and at different ages.

Table 1.6 *Some basal metabolic rate (BMR) values*

Age	Male mass / kg	BMR males / MJ day^{-1}	Female mass / kg	BMR females / MJ day^{-1}
10–18	30	5.0	30	4.6
10–18	65	7.6	60	6.3
19–29	60	6.7	45	4.8
19–29	80	7.9	70	6.4
30–59	65	6.8	50	5.2
30–59	85	7.7	70	5.9

FOOD AND DIET

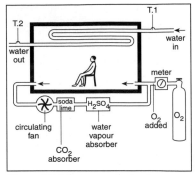

Figure 1.5 A human calorimeter

The differences between the basal metabolic rates in men and women have been attributed to the higher proportion of fatty (adipose) tissue in women. This tissue, although well supplied with blood vessels, is less metabolically active than other body tissues. At rest, when basal metabolic rate is measured, the oxygen uptake is mostly due to the activity of the non-fatty tissues, called the **lean body mass (LBM)**. If the BMR is calculated on the basis of the lean body mass, then it is similar in both sexes.

Basal metabolic rates can be measured by using a human calorimeter, such as the one illustrated in Figure 1.5, which works on the same principles as an ordinary calorimeter, measuring temperature changes over a set period of time.

Alternatively, it can be determined by measuring the uptake of oxygen using a recording spirometer, similar to the one shown in Figure 1.6.

Lean body mass can be calculated from density. It is known that the density of the lean body mass is 1.10, but the density of the whole body is lower, due to the less dense fatty tissues. A thin man will have a density of about 1.075, whereas that of a plump man will be about 1.046. It is difficult to estimate lean body mass directly, as the volume of the body is not easy to measure, but measurements of skinfold thickness can give an indication of the amount of body fat. This can then be deducted from the total body mass to give the lean body mass.

As can be seen from Table 1.6, the BMR varies with age, with body mass and with gender. As age increases, the BMR falls and the decrease is greater for men than for women. The increase in BMR with increase in body mass is to be expected as there is a greater mass of active tissue. The gender differences have already been discussed in relation to the differences in adipose tissue. Other factors which affect the BMR are:
- pregnancy – BMR in females will increase during pregnancy and remain high during lactation
- activity of the thyroid gland – overactivity of the thyroid gland (hyperthyroidism) will cause an increase in the BMR as the hormone thyroxin speeds up the rate at which chemical reactions take place in the body
- disease – fever will cause the BMR to increase by 13 per cent for each °C rise in temperature
- climate – very hot climates cause a reduction of about 10 per cent in the BMR.

As soon as food is eaten, its digestion and absorption leads to an increase in heat production by the body. This is called **diet-induced thermogenesis** and is considered to be caused by the digestive processes and the metabolism of the absorbed food. All food ingestion has this thermic effect and the increase in the BMR is proportional to the energy content of the food eaten.

Having established that the body needs a certain amount of energy to maintain essential internal processes, it is now relevant to consider the variations in energy requirements in relation to daily activities. Any physical activity involves

the use of muscles and the more physical activity undertaken, the greater the amount of energy used up. This energy must be supplied by the diet.
The effect of physical activity on energy requirements is variable. It will depend on:

- the intensity of the activity – some activities, such as swimming, require much more energy (1470 kJ h^{-1}) than others such as riding a bicycle (1030 kJ h^{-1})
- the duration of the activity
- the body size – less energy is required to move a small body mass than a large one.

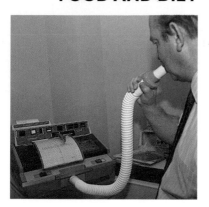

Figure 1.6 Recording spirometer

The energy output and hence the energy requirement of an individual will depend on their occupation and their leisure activities. Different occupations are classified according to whether they are light (sedentary), moderately active or heavy. Working on the assumption that the average person spends 8 hours resting in bed, 8 hours at work and 8 hours on leisure activities, the energy requirements of people in different occupations have been estimated and are shown in Table 1.7.

Table 1.7 *Estimated energy requirements of people in different occupations*

Activity for 8 hours	Sedentary work / MJ per day	Moderately active / MJ per day	Heavy work / MJ per day
resting in bed	2.0	2.0	2.0
at work	4.0	5.5	7.5
leisure	3.0–7.0	3.0–7.0	3.0–7.0
total	9.0–13.0	10.5–14.5	12.5–16.5

Note the range of figures given for the energy needed for leisure activities: this will vary according to the activities chosen.

As already mentioned, energy requirements will vary according to age, gender and body mass. In Table 1.8, the energy requirements of a 35 year old female clerical worker are compared with those of a 25 year old bricklayer, both with a body mass of 60 kg. The bricklayer has moderately active, non-occupational activities, whereas the clerical worker is non-active.

Table 1.8 *Comparison of the energy requirements of a clerical worker and a bricklayer*

Occupation	Gender	Age / years	Body mass / kg	Energy requirement / MJ per day
clerical worker	female	35	60	7.8
bricklayer	male	25	60	12.0

Nutritional requirements vary throughout the lifetime, but at every stage a balanced diet should contain enough energy-giving and growth-promoting foods to satisfy the individual's needs and promote good health. These requirements begin in the uterus during development of the **fetus**. As gestation proceeds, the fetus has an increasing need for all nutrients. There is an increase in the demand for calcium after week 8, as the bones begin to

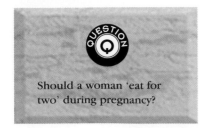

develop, and also iron for the formation of the blood. As the fetus obtains all its nutrients directly from the mother's blood, any factor which reduces her nutrient supply will affect its development.

Once the baby is born, if breast fed, it feeds on milk from its mother. This milk will contain all the nutrients the baby needs in the right quantities and it also has the advantage of being easily digested and absorbed. During the first five days, the milk that is produced, called colostrum at this stage, is rich in antibodies which confer immunity to many illnesses and infections. During **infancy**, the energy and protein requirements continually increase as the child grows in size. There is a continuing need for calcium and vitamin D for the development of strong bones and teeth. In addition, increasing quantities of other vitamins and minerals are needed. There is a need for iron throughout this stage of growth and deficiencies are common. Milk and milk products continue to be valuable sources of protein and calcium in children's diets.

During **puberty**, growth and development is rapid and adolescents often have bigger appetites than adults. The requirements for protein, calcium and iron peak at this stage, as the maximum adult size is reached. The growth spurt, often combined with an increase in physical activity, results in a high demand for energy. Girls begin to menstruate at puberty, so they will have an increased demand for iron. About 20 to 25 mg of iron is lost each month in the menstrual period.

When a woman becomes **pregnant**, a nutrient-dense diet is recommended. The woman does not need to increase her intake of either energy or protein significantly, although it has been estimated that she needs about 1 MJ per day of extra energy. During pregnancy, a woman's protein metabolism and absorption of iron become more efficient. There is, however, an increased demand for certain vitamins and minerals. The requirement for folic acid and calcium almost doubles and that for iron, zinc and iodine also increases. Folic acid is a vitamin, which is required for the formation of DNA in rapidly dividing cells. It is recommended that a woman should increase her intake of folic acid, both pre-conceptually and for the first 12 weeks of a pregnancy. Calcium is needed for the development of bones and teeth in the fetus. Once the baby is born and lactation starts, the requirement for extra nutrients is higher than during pregnancy and the mother needs to ensure that her dietary energy, protein and vitamin intake is high. In addition, she needs to take in extra fluids.

In **old age**, it is still important to eat a balanced diet and to maintain some level of exercise if possible. There may be decreased levels of physical activity if the elderly person is house-bound, so the dietary energy requirements may be reduced, but the need for vitamins and minerals stays the same. Elderly people need a nutrient-dense diet, paying particular attention to the levels of vitamin C, vitamin D and iron. When elderly people live alone, they may eat less fresh food and so may not always obtain enough vitamins and minerals.

Unbalanced diets

If the diet contains less than the required quantities of any particular nutrient or if it contains excessive amounts of nutrients, then it is considered to be unbalanced and thus unhealthy. Both these conditions may lead to serious nutritional disorders if they are allowed to persist.

Undernutrition

Undernutrition can be general, eventually resulting in starvation, or more specifically due to lack of a particular nutrient, such as a vitamin or a mineral ion, which results in a deficiency disease. In general undernutrition, the diet is usually low in energy and protein, giving rise to the deficiency syndrome known as **protein–energy**, or **protein–calorie malnutrition**. This type of malnutrition is common in the poorer countries of the developing world, where protein foods of plant or animal origin may be too expensive or unavailable. Children are more at risk on a low protein diet as their protein requirements are higher than those of adults. Staple foods, such as cassava, may provide some energy, but they contain little protein. They can be supplemented with protein foods, such as pulses, if they are to satisfy the dietary needs. In some cases, a staple such as rice is not sufficiently energy dense and small children cannot eat enough to supply their energy requirements. Where some protein is available, one or more essential (indispensable) amino acids may be lacking. Under these circumstances, body proteins will be used as an energy source and to provide the essential amino acids.

Marasmus and **kwashiorkor** are forms of protein–energy malnutrition which occur, for example, in children in the developing world. About 20 per cent of children in some areas show mild to moderate symptoms of these diseases and a further 2 per cent are severely affected.

Marasmus is caused by early weaning of a child on to a diet which is very low in both energy and protein. It is also associated with poor hygiene, leading to gastrointestinal upsets. The sufferers are grossly underweight, with thin arms and legs, no body fat and show wasting of the muscles. The hair is usually normal, but the face appears old-looking.

Kwashiorkor appears to be linked more with a deficiency of protein in the diet, and develops at a slightly later age than marasmus. In parts of West Africa, young children are weaned on a diet of cassava or green bananas (plantains), usually on the birth of the next child in the family. The carbohydrate content of the diet appears to be adequate, but there is very little protein. This results in symptoms, such as muscle-wasting and swelling (oedema) in the feet and lower legs, pale thin hair and a moon face. The child appears to be miserable and apathetic, and the skin develops patches of pigmentation and becomes flaky. Fat accumulates in the liver and there is a lowering of the blood albumin levels. In severe cases of both marasmus and kwashiorkor, cells in the pancreas and the intestine die, resulting in the reduced production of digestive enzymes and a loss of area over which the absorption of nutrients can occur.

Vitamin deficiencies may be associated with protein–energy malnutrition and a deficiency of **vitamin A (retinol)** is common in children in developing countries. Retinol is a fat-soluble vitamin present in milk, dairy products and fish liver oils. It is not found in plants, but some carotenoids can act as precursors to vitamin A. The β-carotene present in carrots, green leafy vegetables and yellow fruits can be converted to retinol in the wall of the small intestine. This vitamin is needed for the maintenance of healthy epithelial tissues and for the formation of rhodopsin, the visual pigment required for vision at low light intensities. Deficiency of retinol in the diet results initially in night blindness, which may develop into permanent blindness and a condition known as xerophthalmia. Epithelial tissues become keratinised, leading to infections. This deficiency is linked with poverty in the developing world, where diets often lack the expensive animal products, which contain retinol, or dark green leafy vegetables, containing β-carotene which can be converted into retinol in the body.

Vitamin C (ascorbic acid) is needed for the synthesis of collagen and tissue proteins, and it is one of the factors which helps in the absorption of non-haem iron. In addition, it is believed to be involved in the formation of some neurotransmitters in the brain and also with drug detoxification. It is an antioxidant and as such has a protective role in the body by preventing the accumulation of 'free radicals' formed by the spontaneous oxidation of fatty acids. It is a water-soluble vitamin which is easily absorbed, the excess being excreted in the urine. Most animals are able to synthesise their own vitamin C, but primates, including human beings, need to have it supplied in the diet. A deficiency of vitamin C results in **scurvy**, shown by bleeding gums, haemorrhages under the skin and poor wound healing. Because it aids the absorption of non-haem iron, a deficiency may also lead to iron-deficiency anaemia. Good sources of this vitamin in the diet are green vegetables, potatoes and fruit, particularly citrus fruits. Potatoes do not contain large quantities of the vitamin, but make a significant contribution due to the amounts consumed. It is an unstable vitamin, which is destroyed on exposure to high temperatures, oxidation and light. The vitamin C content of foods is reduced on cooking and significant losses take place after harvesting. A diet which does not include fresh vegetables or fruit may be deficient in this vitamin.

Mineral ion deficiencies may also occur. We have already discussed the need for and uptake of **iron** earlier in this chapter. Lack of iron in the diet can result in **iron-deficient anaemia**, which causes general debility, pale appearance and breathlessness. This deficiency is particularly common in women and may occur in infants and young children. In developing countries, the condition may be linked with the occurrence of malaria, where the parasite causes the breakdown of the red blood corpuscles. This results in the release of haemoglobin into the blood plasma: it is broken down and the iron is lost in the urine. The most readily absorbed form of iron is in the haem of haemoglobin, present in red meats, so vegetarians may be at risk of suffering from a deficiency.

Anorexia nervosa and bulimia nervosa

The examples of undernutrition so far discussed have been the result of poor diets, lacking essential nutrients because they are either unavailable or too expensive. Where the eating disorders **anorexia nervosa** and **bulimia nervosa** are concerned, the undernutrition is self-induced.

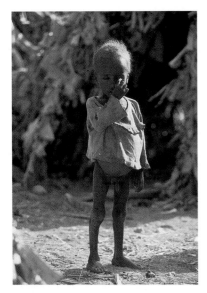

Figure 1.7 A child suffering from marasmus

Anorexia nervosa mainly affects adolescent girls and young women, although it does occur occasionally in young men. The condition starts with dieting to reduce weight, but the dieting may then become so obsessive that the weight loss becomes severe and the body becomes emaciated. In girls, the menstrual periods stop (amenorrhoea) and the sufferer may also have low blood pressure, cold extremities and downy hair. The anorexic person is fearful of becoming fat and will over-estimate the size of their own body. They may show personality changes, a reduction in their social life and act aggressively within the family. The causes are difficult to diagnose, but psychological factors play a significant role, the sufferers often experiencing feelings of inadequacy and an inability to cope with changes taking place at puberty. Once the condition is recognised, recovery, which involves dietary help and psychotherapy, may take as long as two to three years and many sufferers never return to normal eating habits.

Bulimia nervosa involves an irresistible urge to over-eat, or 'binge' on food, followed immediately by self-induced vomiting. Laxatives, diuretics or purgatives may also be used in attempts to prevent weight gain. There may be strict dieting or fasting, as well as vigorous exercising, in between the recurrent episodes of binge eating. The frequent vomiting may lead to a loss of potassium, chloride and hydrogen ions, which will upset the balance of serum electrolytes in the body. Other symptoms include dental erosion, sore throat, swollen salivary glands, fatigue and constipation. Sufferers from bulimia nervosa may not show the extreme weight loss that is characteristic of anorexia nervosa. The condition may develop in people with a history of anorexia nervosa, but bulimia is a distinct disorder and does not occur as a consequence of anorexia nervosa.

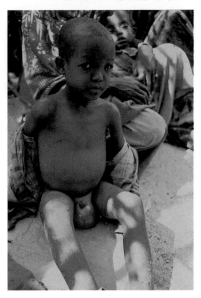

Figure 1.8 A child suffering from kwashiorkor

Overnutrition

Over-nourished people take in more food than they need and may become **overweight** or **obese**. It has been estimated that, in the UK, about 60 per cent of men and 40 per cent of women are overweight or **obese**. Overweight people are more susceptible to illness as they become older.

It is relevant here to define what is meant by 'overweight' and to distinguish between that term and obesity. An obese person has an excessive amount of body fat. In everyone, a certain proportion of the body mass is composed of fatty (adipose) tissue. There is a subcutaneous layer, necessary for insulation, and there is adipose tissue around the kidneys and other organs. In men, it is acceptable that between 12 per cent and 17 per cent of the body weight is made up of fatty tissue. In women, this proportion rises slightly to between 20 per cent and 25 per cent. It is useful to be able to assess whether or not a person is underweight, overweight or obese, and to do this the height and body mass are used to calculate a **body mass index (BMI)**. The body mass, in kg, is divided by the height, in metres, squared.

$$\text{BMI} = \frac{\text{body mass}}{(\text{height})^2}$$

So, the BMI of a person with a body mass of 65 kg and height 1.72 m would be 21.78. Reference to Table 1.9 will indicate to which category the person belongs. The figure falls between 20 and 24.9, which is considered to be normal.

Table 1.9 *The use of Body Mass Index (BMI) to classify body weight*

Body Mass Index (BMI)	Description of body weight
below 20	underweight
20–24.9	normal
25–29.9	overweight
30–40	moderately obese
over 40	severely obese

It is very difficult to determine exactly what causes obesity. We know that an obese person has a greater proportion of adipose tissue than a normal person and we also know that weight gain will occur only if the energy content of a person's diet exceeds their energy expenditure. The excess energy intake is stored as fat. It is also known that excessive alcohol consumption can contribute to weight gain, because alcohol has a high energy content. Overweight people do not necessarily eat more than people with a normal weight – very often they eat less. As there is much interest in controlling obesity, several factors which might cause it have been considered. These include:

- metabolic factors – do fat people have a different metabolism from thin people? The BMR of obese people may be higher than that of people of normal weight. The results of studies on metabolic rates and the thermic response to extra food in the diet suggest that there are differences in the way that food energy is used by different individuals and that overeating does not result in similar degrees of weight gain.

- the nature of the food in the diet – are some foods more fattening than others? There does not appear to be any evidence to suggest that any particular food can promote weight loss or weight gain. Obviously it is important to control the proportions of energy-dense and nutrient-dense foods in the diet in order to promote or prevent changes in weight.

- levels of physical activity – reducing physical activity in people who are overweight may contribute to weight gain, but there does not seem to be much evidence to support the idea that low levels of physical activity on their own cause obesity.

- eating behaviour – the more palatable the food, the more of it we are likely to eat, whether we need it or not. Experiments with rats have shown that they will overeat if given free access to palatable foods. The reasons for eating food, apart from satisfying our daily nutritional requirements, are complex, but it has been observed that overweight people tend to underestimate the quantities of food that they consume.

- genetic factors – do we inherit a predisposition to obesity? It is difficult to separate out any genetic influence from all the other factors, but studies have indicated that there is some correlation between the BMIs of parents and their offspring. However, the recent rapid increase in obesity is unlikely to be due to a change in the gene pool, so it may be that overeating is learned by offspring from their parents.

- hormonal factors – these do not appear to cause obesity, but hormonal abnormalities are more likely to result from obesity. For example, overweight people are more likely to develop Type 2 (maturity onset) diabetes than people of normal weight.

- psychological factors – it has been suggested that overeating leading to obesity is a form of stress-induced behaviour. It has even been proposed that some people develop an addiction to carbohydrates in the same way as they might develop an addiction to drugs or alcohol.

Obese people have a higher mortality rate than people of normal weight. It has been estimated that a BMI of 35 causes the mortality rate to be twice that for people of the same age with a BMI of between 20 and 25. Obesity has been shown to be a contributory or causative factor in a number of different conditions. These include:
- coronary heart disease
- hypertension (increased blood pressure)
- mature onset diabetes
- an increased risk of osteoarthritis, especially of the knees, hips and spine
- an increased risk of complications during surgery
- infertility in women
- gall bladder disease – especially in women
- difficulties in childbirth in women
- an increased risk of developing toxaemia during pregnancy
- an increased risk of breast, cervical and uterine cancer in women
- an increased risk of cancer of the colon, rectum and prostate gland in men.

In view of these many and varied effects, the treatment of obesity is important. The main objective of any treatment is to reduce the amount of energy intake, especially from fat, whilst increasing the amount of energy expenditure by the body. Basically, this means eating less and doing more exercise. But it is not quite as simple as that, because the amount of energy expended on quite vigorous exercise is low. However, regular exercise will tone the body and help to stimulate greater diet-induced thermogenesis (heat production in response to food intake).

Ideally, weight loss should be gradual and the overweight person should recognise the benefits of making permanent dietary changes in order that, once any diet has been stopped, their weight does not increase again. Crash diets, which cut down drastically on the quantity of food consumed, are dangerous to general health, because important nutrients will be lacking. Very low calorie diets have been popular because they lead to rapid weight loss, but they may produce unpleasant side-effects such as diarrhoea and nausea. If continued for long periods, such diets could result in deficiency symptoms. In addition, such drastic dieting does not result in a change in eating habits. The best strategy is a diet which is low in energy and fat with a high nutrient density, combined with an active lifestyle.

2 Diet and health

Foods are organic and provide a range of nutrients for microorganisms, which may cause spoilage. In this chapter, we consider a range of additives, substances which are added to foods for a variety of purposes, including the prevention of spoilage. The relationships between diet and health are considered, including possible risk factors in coronary heart disease. Contamination of food by microorganisms, which results in food poisoning, is also described.

Additives

For centuries, humans have used a range of food additives, mainly as preservatives to increase the time for which food can be kept in a palatable condition. Unless treated in some way, numerous different microorganisms, including bacteria and fungi, will grow on foods, resulting in spoilage and increasing the risk of food poisoning. Cereal grains, such as wheat and barley, are an exception to this and, if kept dry, will last for years without deteriorating. Examples of microorganisms which cause food spoilage are shown in Table 2.1.

Table 2.1 *Examples of microorganisms which cause spoilage of fresh foods*

Food types	Types of microorganisms	Examples which cause spoilage
fruit and vegetables	bacteria	*Erwinia, Pseudomonas*
	fungi	*Aspergillus, Rhizopus, Penicillium*
fresh meat, including poultry and seafood	bacteria	*Escherichia, Proteus, Pseudomonas, Salmonella*
	fungi	*Mucor, Penicillium, Rhizopus*
milk	bacteria	*Lactobacillus, Streptococcus*

Food additives are substances which are added in small amounts to processed foods for a specific purpose. The Food Labelling Regulations (1984) define an additive as:

'any substance not commonly regarded or used as a food, which is added to or used in or on food at any stage to affect its keeping qualities, texture, consistency, appearance, taste, odour, alkalinity or acidity or to serve any other technological function in relation to food.'

Only substances which are known as permitted additives may be used in food. Most permitted additives have been allocated a serial number; where the use of that additive is also controlled by the European Union (EU), the number is prefixed by an E-. Some additives are permitted in the United Kingdom and some other countries, but are not covered by EU legislation. These have numbers without the E- prefix.

Table 2.2 *Some examples of permitted food additives*

E-numbers	Category	Examples
E-100 to E-180	colouring materials	E-102 tartrazine
E-200 to E-290	preservatives	E-211 sodium benzoate
E-300 to E-322	antioxidants	E-300 ascorbic acid
E-400 to E-483	emulsifiers and stabilisers	E-412 guar gum

Additives can be classified into two main groups: those which prevent spoilage, and those which are added to improve the flavour, texture, or appearance of the food. Examples of the major types of food additives and their uses are shown in Table 2.3.

Rancidity is the most common form of chemical spoilage of food, resulting from the oxidation of fats and oils by atmospheric oxygen. This can be reduced by the addition of antioxidants. The development of rancid 'off' flavours results from the reaction of long-chain fatty acids, containing two or more double bonds, to form short-chain fatty acids. These resulting short-chain fatty acids, such as butyric acid, impart unpleasant flavours to the food.

Colouring agents may be added to foods to return the food to its original colour if this has been changed or lost during processing. The appearance of foods can be enhanced by the addition of colouring agents – people expect foods to look appetising, and to be the appropriate colour, as well as tasting good. Some examples of colouring agents and their corresponding E-numbers are shown in Table 2.4. Flavouring agents, or flavours, are added to increase the attractiveness of foods and may be used in food without restrictions. There are thousands of different flavourings available for use in food. These include natural substances, such as herbs, spices and essential oils, and a range of synthetic substances including esters, ethers and alcohols. Many artificial fruit flavours are esters, formed by the reaction between alcohols and organic acids. These fruit-flavoured esters are the most widely used types of flavourings, some of which are shown in Table 2.5.

It is a legal requirement that certain nutrients are added to white flour and to margarine. Flour is produced in a process known as **milling**, in which grains of wheat are crushed by passing them through a series of rollers. The percentage of flour produced from the wheat is known as the extraction rate of the flour; wholemeal flour, which contains all parts of the wheat grain, has an extraction rate of 100 per cent. Flour millers are required by law (Bread and Flour Regulations, 1995), to add nutrients to all flour, other than wholemeal flour, as vitamins and minerals are lost during the milling process. Nutrients are added to ensure that the concentrations of these correspond to those which occur naturally in flour with an extraction rate of 80 per cent. Sufficient iron, thiamin, niacin and purified chalk (calcium carbonate) must be added to ensure that 100 g of the flour will contain not less than:

- 1.6 g iron
- 0.24 mg thiamin
- 1.60 mg niacin
- between 235 and 390 mg calcium carbonate.

The Spreadable Fats (Marketing Standards) Regulations, 1995, include the requirements for vitamins A and D in margarine. These vitamins occur naturally in milk and dairy products, such as butter, but the concentration varies during the year, being highest during the summer when cows are eating fresh grass. Vitamins A and D are added to margarine so that it contains 800 to 1000 μg of vitamin A (retinol equivalent) per 100 g and 7 to 9 μg vitamin D per 100 g. This means that margarine will have a vitamin content which is equal to that of summer butter. These vitamins may also be added to dairy spreads which contain butter, but this is not essential.

Table 2.3 *Examples of food additives and some of their uses*

Food additives	Examples	Functions
antioxidants	ascorbic acid, propyl gallate, butylated hydroxyanisole (BHA), tocopherols	used to prevent oxidation of fats and oils by atmospheric oxygen, resulting in the development of rancid flavours
anti-caking agents	calcium hydroxy phosphate, magnesium carbonate	prevent the formation of lumps in powdery foods such as icing sugar and powdered milk
colours	natural – β-carotene, chlorophyll synthetic – tartrazine, erythrosine	mainly used to make food products look attractive to the consumer
emulsifiers	lecithins	used to prevent the separation of oils and water in, for example, sauces and soft margarines
food acids	citric acid, acetic acid	used for flavouring or to control setting in jam; also used as preservatives
flavour enhancers	monosodium glutamate, sodium inosinate	used to enhance the taste or smell of food without giving any flavour of their own
humectants	glycerol, sorbitol	prevent food, such as royal icing, from drying out and becoming hard and unpalatable
nutritional supplements	vitamins A, D, B_{12}, nicotinic acid	a number of foods are enriched with vitamins; as examples, margarine contains vitamins A and D, breakfast cereals contain some B vitamins
preservatives	sorbic acid, sulphur dioxide, sodium metabisulphite	inhibit the growth of bacteria and fungi in foods and therefore prevent microbial spoilage
sweeteners	sorbitol, mannitol, saccharin, aspartame, acesulpham-K	used to impart a sweet flavour to foods and drinks; used in low-calorie products
thickeners	guar gum, pectin, alginates, carboxy methylcellulose	increase the viscosity of foods; used in a wide range of products such as packet cheesecake mixes, sauces, ice cream and instant desserts

Table 2.4 *Some examples of food colouring agents*

Colouring substance	E-number	Colour
amaranth	E-123	red
beta-carotene	E-160(a)	yellow/orange
caramel	E-150	brown
erythrosine BS	E-127	red
lycopene	E-160(d)	red
tartrazine	E-120	yellow

Table 2.5 *Some examples of esters used as flavouring agents*

Name	Uses
allyl caproate	pineapple essence
ethyl acetate	apple, pear, strawberry and peach essences
ethyl formate	rum, raspberry and peach essences
pentyl acetate	pear, pineapple and raspberry essences

As an example to illustrate the uses of food additives, the following list of ingredients is taken from a carton of gravy granules:

Hydrogenated vegetable oil, starch, salt, wheat flour, dried onion, hydrolysed vegetable protein, colour (E150), sugar, flavour enhancers (E621, E635), emulsifier (lecithin, (E322)), yeast extract, herb and spice extracts.

Sugars and sweeteners

Substances such as sugars, starches, cellulose, pectins, gums and mucilages are all carbohydrates. Simple sugars, including glucose and fructose, are found in honey and various fruits. These simple sugars are often mixed with disaccharides, such as sucrose, found in sugar beet and sugar cane. The chemical nature, occurrence, digestion and absorption of sugars have already been described; in this section we look at sweetness and the uses of artificial sweeteners.

Not all sugars have a sweet taste and the degree of sweetness varies widely. Sucrose is used as the standard reference substance for sweetness, having a threshold concentration (minimum concentration which produces a response on the tongue) of 0.01 mol dm^{-3}. The degree of sweetness of different sugars is usually compared with that of sucrose, which has been assigned a relative sweetness (RS) of 1.0. As it is not possible to say with certainty that a substance is so many times sweeter than sucrose, relative sweetness is determined by finding the concentration of the substance which can be tasted. **Relative sweetness** is then calculated from this concentration relative to the threshold for sucrose.

Fructose is sweeter tasting than sucrose, but glucose, maltose and lactose are less sweet than sucrose. The relative sweetness of various sweeteners, both natural and artificial, is shown in Table 2.6.

Thousands of sweet-tasting substances have been identified, including a wide range of chemical classes, but only about 20 are permitted for use in food. As far as legislation is concerned, the common food sugars and glucose syrups are not considered to be sweeteners. Artificial sweeteners are classified as either bulk sweeteners or intense sweeteners. Bulk sweeteners are generally less sweet tasting than sucrose, but intense sweeteners may be thousands of times sweeter than sucrose. Intense sweeteners are useful in the formulation of low-calorie food products, but many have the disadvantage of unpleasant aftertastes, such as bitterness or a metallic taste. Bulk sweeteners taste very similar to sucrose, but have similar calorific values. They do, however, have advantages including stability in solution, and may be used in confectionery, rendering it less harmful to teeth. Bulk and intense sweeteners are sometimes

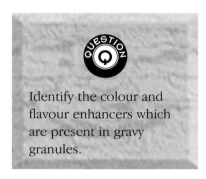

Identify the colour and flavour enhancers which are present in gravy granules.

Table 2.6 *Relative sweetness of various sweeteners*

Sweetener	Relative sweetness
sucrose	1.0
fructose	1.73
glucose	0.74
honey	0.97
sorbitol	0.5
aspartame	200
saccharin	300

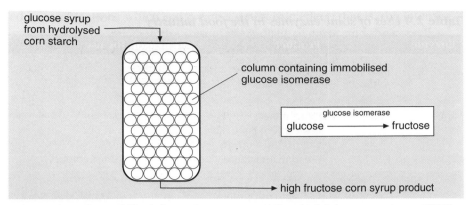

Figure 2.1 Use of immobilised glucose isomerase to produce high fructose corn syrup (HFCS) in a continuous process

Amyloglucosidase (glucoamylase) is an enzyme which catalyses the hydrolysis of 1,4- and 1,6-alpha-linkages in starch, removing glucose units stepwise from one end of the substrate molecule. Amyloglucosidase is used to produce high glucose syrups from corn starch. The glucose syrups are then used directly in a range of food and drinks, including fruit sorbets, and as a substrate for the production of fructose syrups, using glucose isomerase. Amyloglucosidase can also be used in an immobilised preparation and will remain active for up to 100 hours at 60 °C.

Other enzymes used in the food industry include **lactase** and **proteases**. Lactase is used in the manufacture of low-lactose milk. Sterilised, skimmed milk is passed through a column containing beads of immobilised lactase, which breaks down the lactose present in milk to glucose and galactose. This makes milk acceptable to those with **lactose intolerance**, which is described in Chapter 1.

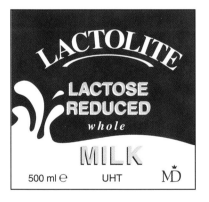

Figure 2.2(b) Lactolite – lactose reduced milk

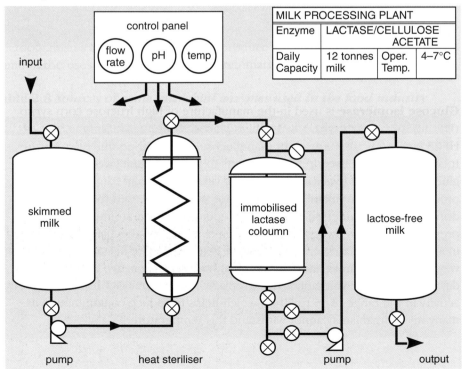

Figure 2.2 (a) Industrial production of lactose free milk;

Proteases have a number of applications in the food industry including meat tenderisation, manufacture of cheese, and softening of bread dough. Meat tenderisation is increased using enzymes obtained from plant sources, including papain and bromelain, or from microbial sources. The role of rennin in the production of cheese is described in Chapter 4.

Concerns about additives

Concern has been expressed about possible adverse effects on consumers due to the presence of additives in foods. However, it is generally agreed that using food additives is justified if they fulfil one or more of the following functions:
- maintenance of nutritional quality
- improvement of keeping quality with less wastage
- making the food product look more attractive, without being deceptive.

Additives should never be used, for example, to disguise faulty handling or processing, or to deceive the consumer. It is essential that any risks of possible side-effects from the presence of additives in food should be negligible when compared with the corresponding benefits. Food additives approved for use in Britain have useful functions and cause no harm to the vast majority of consumers. Nevertheless, some people who are sensitive to food additives are sensitive to substances naturally present in foods, and may have adverse reactions. In a food allergy, the body's immune system responds to certain harmless substances present in food. As a result, **histamine** is released, from basophils and mast cells, into the bloodstream. This results in a series of symptoms including swelling of the lips, urticaria (nettle rash), asthma, headache, vomiting and diarrhoea. The food additives commonly associated with food allergies include tartrazine and benzoates (used as preservatives in a range of products including jam, pickles and coffee essence).

Ben Finegold, a doctor working in the USA, suggested that hyperactivity in children, usually boys, would be reduced if they were fed on a diet which cut out all food and drink containing certain additives. These include synthetic colourings and flavourings, nitrates, nitrites, butyulated hydroxyanisole (BHA), butylated hydroxytoluene (BHT) and benzoic acid. Foods containing natural salicylates, including almonds, apricots, plums, oranges, tomatoes and raisins, should also be avoided for four to six weeks, then re-introduced in the diet one at a time, to see whether there are any adverse effects. Although this approach has some support, there is little clinical evidence to confirm a link between additives and behavioural disorders. A study carried out at Great Ormond Street Hospital did, however, show that some children with a combination of hyperactivity and physical symptoms including rashes and headaches, improved on an elimination diet. These children appeared to be particularly sensitive to tartrazine and benzoic acid. As a result of concern about possible adverse effects of tartrazine, manufacturers usually avoid this in their products.

Additives which are intentionally added to foods are not harmful; they have all been thoroughly tested and are continually monitored for any adverse effects. The amounts of additives which are allowed in foods are such that the maximum intake does not exceed 1/100 of the highest concentration which has no effects in animal tests.

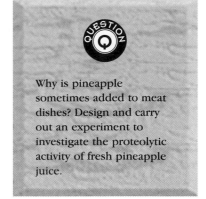

Why is pineapple sometimes added to meat dishes? Design and carry out an experiment to investigate the proteolytic activity of fresh pineapple juice.

Table 2.10 *Foods which are likely to contain tartrazine (E-120)*

cakes	marmalade
custard	yoghurt
fizzy drinks	ice cream
fruit squashes	jelly
packet and tinned soups	mustard
pickles	ice lollies
salad cream	jam
sweets	marzipan

Coronary heart disease

Coronary heart disease and the associated risk factors are described in Chapter 2 of *Systems and their Maintenance*. There are a number of different factors associated with coronary heart disease, including family history of heart disease, increased plasma cholesterol, diabetes, high blood pressure, smoking and obesity, but diet is probably the most important environmental factor. The basis of coronary heart disease is the formation of arteriosclerosis, a descriptive term for hardening, thickening and loss of elasticity of blood-vessel walls. The most common type of arteriosclerosis affects the large and medium-sized arteries, in which there is an underlying abnormal change in the vessel wall known as **atheroma**. This type of arteriosclerosis is, therefore, known as **atherosclerosis**. Accumulation of lipids and other changes in the structure of the vessel wall result in the formation of a raised **atheromatous plaque**, which narrows the lumen of the artery and obstructs blood flow. This type of atheroma occurs commonly in the coronary artery of cigarette-smoking males. A frequent symptom of this narrowing of the coronary artery is a condition known as angina pectoris, a pain in the chest, particularly following exertion and settling with rest. Further narrowing of the lumen of the coronary artery can abruptly reduce blood flow to the heart muscle which becomes deprived of oxygen resulting in tissue death. This death, or necrosis, of an area of cardiac muscle is known as myocardial infarction, often referred to as a heart attack.

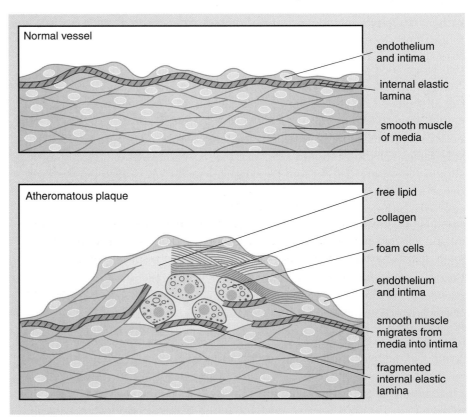

Figure 2.3 The formation of an atheromatous plaque

The factors which are likely to lead to severe atherosclerosis are now well-recognised and can be divided into three main groups:
- constitutional factors, including age, sex and genetic factors
- 'hard risk' factors, including high plasma cholesterol concentration, high blood pressure and smoking
- 'soft risk' factors, such as lack of regular exercise, obesity and stressful lifestyle.

The material which accumulates in atherosclerosis is cholesterol, which is transported in the blood, associated with lipoproteins (low density lipoproteins, LDL). The risk of coronary heart disease increases steadily with increased plasma cholesterol. Many investigations have shown that people with plasma cholesterol concentrations higher than 6.5 mmol dm^{-3} are at high risk; people with plasma cholesterol concentrations between 5.2 mmol dm^{-3} and 6.5 mmol dm^{-3} are at moderate risk.

The main dietary influence on plasma LDL and cholesterol is the amount and type of fat in food. Polyunsaturated fats, particularly linoleic acid, tend to lower plasma LDL and total cholesterol. Other dietary factors associated with coronary heart disease include **non-starch polysaccharides** (dietary fibre) and possibly **salt** (sodium chloride). The effect of non-starch polysaccharides depends on the type. Insoluble forms, such as cellulose, do not decrease plasma cholesterol, but soluble types, including pectins and gums, may help to reduce plasma cholesterol. Soluble non-starch polysaccharides are present in oatmeal, beans, fruit and vegetables. High salt intake probably causes high blood pressure, but the evidence supporting this is not clear. Nevertheless, it is recommended that the salt intake should not exceed 6 g per day.

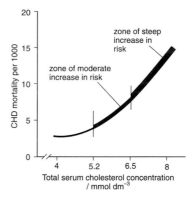

Figure 2.4 The relationship between total cholesterol and risk of coronary heart disease based on a six year study of over 350 000 middle-aged men in the United States

Diseases of the colon

The chemical nature, sources and importance of non-starch polysaccharides (NSP) are described in Chapter 1. The laxative effect of NSP is generally well known, but dietary NSP is important in several other aspects of health, including **constipation, cancer of the large intestine, diverticular disease** and **irritable bowel syndrome**. Diets rich in the soluble forms of NSP may help to lower blood cholesterol levels, which may, in turn, reduce the incidence of coronary heart disease. Malignant tumours of the colon and rectum are very common, particularly in Western countries, and are the second largest cause of death from cancer. It has been shown that wheat fibre, fruit and vegetables may offer some protection. Epidemiological studies have shown that that stool weights below 150 g per day are associated with an increased risk of bowel cancer. NSP decreases the transit time which reduces the time for which any potentially carcinogenic substance is in contact with the mucosa of the intestine.

Non-starch polysaccharides, which are not digested in the human stomach or small intestine, reach the colon where they are fermented by bacteria. This process produces a number of substances, including short-chain fatty acids such as butyrate. Butyrate has been shown to regulate cell growth in the large intestine and may help to prevent cells in the colon from developing into a cancer.

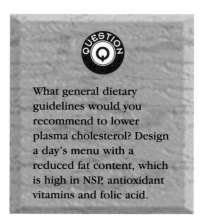

What general dietary guidelines would you recommend to lower plasma cholesterol? Design a day's menu with a reduced fat content, which is high in NSP, antioxidant vitamins and folic acid.

Diverticular disease and constipation are both common in the elderly, although thay can occur at any age, and are found predominantly in the Western hemisphere. Diverticular disease arises as increased pressure within the colon results in the formation of 'pouches' of the mucosa which project through areas of the circular muscle layer. It is possible that this results from abnormally high pressure in the colon associated with low NSP diets. Irritable bowel syndrome is a condition involving the small and large intestine and is characterised by abdominal pain, constipation or diarrhoea, and nausea. There is some evidence that this is caused by sensitivity to certain foods, including dairy products, maize, some fruits, tea and coffee. It is important to ensure enough NSP in the diet to promote regular bowel habit.

Dietary aspects of diabetes mellitus

Diabetes mellitus is one of the most common disorders of the endocrine system and affects about 1.4 million people in the UK (1996). In people with diabetes, an inadequate amount of insulin may be produced. In some other affected people, decreased numbers of insulin receptors on the target cells make it impossible for glucose to be taken up by these cells even if insulin is present. Insulin, which is produced by the β cells of the pancreatic islets, increases the uptake of glucose, fatty acids and amino acids, from the blood and into tissue cells. Consequently, insulin decreases the blood concentrations of these substances and promotes their metabolism by tissue cells, chiefly skeletal muscle, adipose tissue and liver. In diabetes mellitus, glucose cannot enter cells normally and the result is an increase in blood glucose concentrations, a condition known as hyperglycaemia. The normal resting levels of glucose in the blood are between 4.5 and 5.5 mmol dm^{-3}, but in hyperglycaemia the resting blood glucose concentrations may rise to 11 mmol dm^{-3}, and up to 28 mmol dm^{-3} following a meal. Glucose will be filtered out of the blood in the kidneys, but the rate of appearance of glucose in the filtrate will exceed the rate at which glucose can be reabsorbed. As a consequence, glucose appears in the urine. Glucose remaining in the filtrate has an osmotic effect, resulting in larger than normal volumes of urine being produced, with consequent dehydration and feelings of thirst. In untreated diabetes, cells are unable to use glucose as a substrate for respiration, so substances such as amino acids and fatty acids are used instead.

If glucose metabolism is severely reduced, metabolism of large quantities of fatty acids produces toxic by-products known collectively as **ketone bodies**. A build up of these substances reduces the pH of the blood from 7.4 to 7.0, resulting in a condition referred to as **diabetic ketoacidosis**. Symptoms of this include abdominal pain, nausea, a 'fruity' (pear-drops) odour of the breath, unconsciousness, coma and, if untreated, may lead to death.

There are two main types of diabetes mellitus, known as **type I** and **type II**. Type I diabetes mellitus is also referred to as **juvenile onset diabetes**, because it usually occurs before the age of 40. In this form of diabetes, secretion of insulin is very low, or absent. People with type I diabetes are required to take regular injections of insulin to control hyperglycaemia and prevent ketoacidosis. Type I diabetes is, therefore, also known as insulin dependent diabetes.

Type II diabetes, or non-insulin dependent diabetes, is the most common form of this disorder and accounts for about 90 per cent of all cases. This type occurs most often after the age of 40 and is, therefore, also known as **mature onset diabetes**. In this form of diabetes, insulin is still produced by the β cells, but loss of insulin receptors on the cell surface membranes of target cells may reduce the uptake of glucose from the blood. The development of type II diabetes is closely associated with obesity (Figure 2.5), although hereditary factors are also important. In type II diabetes, injection of insulin may not be required and hyperglycaemia can be controlled by eating a balanced diet, taking adequate exercise and maintaining body weight within normal limits.

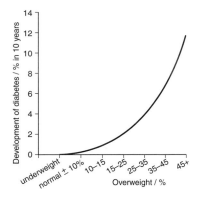

Figure 2.5 *The relationship between body weight and subsequent development of diabetes*

The British Diabetic Association recommends that diets for diabetics should contain:
* at least 50 per cent of calories as carbohydrates, mostly from foods high in starch
* about 30 to 35 per cent of calories as fats, with saturated fats restricted to 10 per cent.

In type I diabetes, the emphasis should be on foods which are low in fat and have a low glycaemic index, such as lentils and other legumes, pasta, All Bran, cherries, apples, oranges and peaches. Diets which are high in non-starch polysaccharides (NSP) have also proved to be helpful to diabetics. In particular, the soluble forms of NSP are able to reduce the rate of uptake of glucose from the gut into the bloodstream.

People with diabetes are advised to:
* eat regular meals and eat similar amounts of starchy foods from day to day
* eat foods which are high in NSP, especially beans, peas, lentils, vegetables, fruit and oats
* cut down on fried and fatty foods including butter, margarine, cheese and fatty meat
* reduce intake of sugar by replacing high-sugar foods, such as tinned fruits in syrup, for low sugar foods
* drink alcohol in moderation only

Food poisoning

The term **food poisoning** is widely used to describe a range of infections of the gastrointestinal tract. These can be caused by a number of different microorganisms, including bacteria and viruses, which are acquired as a result of the consumption of contaminated food or water. Bacteria are widely present in the environment, including soil, air and water. The majority of them are harmless, but some, referred to as **pathogenic bacteria**, or **pathogens**, can cause disease.

Food can become contaminated with pathogenic bacteria in a variety of different ways. Meat, and meat products, may be contaminated as a result of coming from animals which were already hosts to the bacteria. Many cases of food poisoning may be the result of unhygienic human behaviour, or inappropriate food handling and processing. People handling food may themselves be infected with a microorganism which causes food poisoning and yet have no symptoms so that they are unaware of the infection. These people are known as carriers, and can spread infection from person to person, usually by means of contaminated food or water. In one well-known example, 'Typhoid Mary', a cook working in New York in the 1900's, was a carrier of *Salmonella* and was responsible for starting at least 20 outbreaks of typhoid.

Animals may also harbour food-poisoning microorganisms and can spread them to humans by coming into contact with food. Examples of such animals are rats, mice, cockroaches, domestic pets and wild birds. Many pathogens which cause food poisoning are spread by means of faeces, from animals or humans, which may contaminate food or water.

In order for infection to occur, the pathogenic organisms must be ingested in sufficient numbers and be able to avoid destruction by the body's immune system. When the pathogens reach the intestines, they cause disease as a result of multiplication and/or by toxin production, or they may invade the mucosa of the intestine to reach the lymphatic system or bloodstream. Food poisoning may also occur as a result of the consumption of food containing toxins produced by bacteria, which multiply within the contaminated food. As an example, the bacterium *Bacillus cereus*, which is common in soil, dust, cereals and many other foods, produces a heat-stable toxin which causes vomiting within 1 to 5 hours of ingestion of contaminated food, commonly reheated, cooked rice. *Bacillus cereus* can produce spores which are resistant to boiling but will grow and produce toxins at a suitable temperature.

Infections of the gastrointestinal tract range in their effects from mild to severe, and sometimes fatal, diarrhoea. This may be associated with vomiting, fever, flu-like symptoms and abdominal pain. Some of the bacteria which cause food poisoning, and their sources of infection, are shown in Table 2.11.

Table 2.11 *Some causes and sources of bacterial food poisoning*

Organism	Sources of infection
Bacillus cereus	commonly associated with reheated, cooked rice and pulses
Campylobacter jejuni	infected foods, especially poultry, milk and water; consumption of milk from bottles with tops pecked by wild birds
Escherichia coli	*E. coli* is normally present in the gut, but there are a number of pathogenic strains which can cause diarrhoeal diseases; spread by contact with faeces and contaminated water, raw or inadequately cooked poultry and meat
Listeria monocytogenes	found in a wide range of foods, including milk, certain soft cheeses, pre-cooked meat and pâté
Salmonella enteritidis	raw or inadequately cooked meat, milk, eggs, or poultry
Staphylococcus aureus	cold meats and poultry, trifles and cream products. *Staphylococcus aureus* is normally present on the skin, especially in the nose and around the anus. It produces a toxin which results in severe vomiting within 3 to 6 hours of consumption of contaminated food

It can be seen from Table 2.11 that certain foods are particularly likely to become contaminated with pathogenic bacteria if not handled, stored, or cooked properly. These are referred to as **high-risk foods** and include:

- cooked meats and cooked meat products
- milk, cream, custard and dairy produce
- shellfish
- cooked rice
- eggs and egg products.

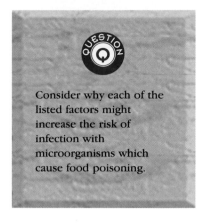

Consider why each of the listed factors might increase the risk of infection with microorganisms which cause food poisoning.

The number of reported cases of food poisoning in England and Wales now exceeds 40 000 per year, but as many cases may go unreported, the total incidence is probably considerably higher than this. There are a number of reasons why there are so many cases of what is essentially a preventable disease, including:

- increased use of convenience foods, which may be inadequately cooked at home
- increased consumption of take-away meals
- increased communal feeding, varied menus and fast-food service which can affect large numbers of people if the food is contaminated
- changing patterns of shopping and food storage in the home.

To illustrate how modern methods of food handling and processing have contributed to the incidence of food poisoning, we will consider contamination of foods by *Salmonella enteriditis* and *Listeria monocytogenes*. Until recently, infection with *Salmonella* was the most common cause of food-associated diarrhoea in the western world. In some countries, however, this has now been overtaken by infection with *Campylobacter*. The genus *Salmonella* has been divided into more than 2000 species, but it is now considered that these are different varieties of three species, *Salmonella cholerae-suis, S. typhi*, and *S. enteriditis. Salmonella* occurs widely among animals; chickens often act as carriers and eggs may become infected either from bacteria present in the oviduct of a hen, or through contamination by chicken droppings after the eggs are laid. Since 1987 there has been an increase in the number of cases of food poisoning due to *Salmonella enteriditis*, particularly from raw eggs, lightly cooked eggs, or products containing raw egg such as mayonnaise or home-made ice cream.

Infection with *Salmonella enteriditis* causes diarrhoea within six hours to two days. People who have been infected with *Salmonella* may carry and continue to excrete organisms in their faeces for up to two months, so it is essential to wash the hands properly before handling food to prevent spread. Because there is a large reservoir of *Salmonella* in animals, it is impossible to eliminate the bacteria entirely; control measures are therefore aimed at breaking the chain between animals and humans, and between humans.

Listeria monocytogenes is a species of bacterium which has widespread occurrence in both animals and the environment. Humans may also carry *Listeria* as part of the normal intestinal flora. It can survive long periods of drying and freezing, and can multiply in foods kept at 4 °C. It is of particular

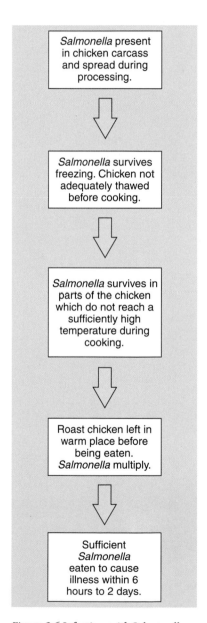

Figure 2.6 Infection with Salmonella *from inadequately cooked poultry*

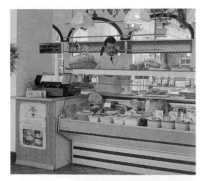

Figure 2.7 A delicatessen counter in a supermarket showing a range of cheeses and cooked meats

concern therefore in cook–chill foods – those which have been processed or heated and are then kept in cold storage to be sold as ready-to-eat, such as sandwiches, dairy produce, pies and cold meats.

Listeria may be present in domestic animals, including cows, and is present in large numbers in the milk of infected cows. Infection of *Listeria* in humans causes the disease known as listeriosis, which is particularly dangerous to pregnant women. The symptoms may be similar to those of a mild, flu-like illness, but the infection can cause spontaneous abortion or premature birth of the baby, which may itself be infected. Infection of the fetus can result in stillbirth, or serious, often fatal, disease of the new-born baby. The disease can also occur in other adults, particularly those with an impaired immune system, and the elderly, who develop symptoms of meningitis which can be fatal.

Pregnant women are advised to wash fruit and vegetables thoroughly and not to eat certain uncooked foods which are considered to be of particular risk, such as unpasteurised milk, cheeses made from unpasteurised milk, coleslaw and pâté.

Prevention of food poisoning

In order to help prevent food poisoning, it is important to prevent contamination of foods with pathogenic microorganisms and to maintain conditions which will halt or reduce their growth. In particular it is important to:

- cook food thoroughly. Cooking times and temperatures must be sufficient to destroy all bacteria and their toxins. Some bacterial spores may not be destroyed by boiling
- eat cooked food within one hour of cooking
- never freeze or re-heat food more than once
- keep foods at an appropriate temperature. Refrigerate at less than 4 °C
- keep raw and cooked foods separate during storage and preparation
- use only fresh eggs stored in a refrigerator and use before the 'best by' date
- defrost meat and poultry thoroughly before cooking, then cook thoroughly until the juices run clear

- use separate knives and other utensils for raw and cooked food
- ensure high standards of personal hygiene. Wash hands thoroughly and dry using clean towels, disposable paper towels or a hot air drier
- thoroughly clean surfaces and utensils which have come into contact with raw foods
- keep animals, including pets, away from food preparation areas.

Other diseases spread via contaminated food and water

The ingestion of pathogenic microorganisms in contaminated food or water can cause many different infections. So far in this chapter we have concentrated mainly on those which are associated with food poisoning and gastrointestinal symptoms, but infections acquired via the gastrointestinal tract can cause diseases in other body systems, if the microorganisms are able to invade the mucous surface of the intestine and spread to other tissues These diseases include some forms of viral hepatitis, typhoid fever, listeriosis and botulism. The causes and symptoms of certain other diseases which are acquired from contaminated food or water are shown in Table 2.12.

Table 2.12 *Causes and symptoms of some diseases which are acquired through contaminated food or water*

Disease	Causative organisms	Symptoms
dysentery	*Shigella* spp. including *S. dysenteriae*, a Gram-negative, rod-shaped bacterium; dysentery may also be caused by a number of protozoa, including *Entamoeba histolytica*	Inflammation of the gastrointestinal tract, often associated with blood and pus in the faeces; diarrhoea, pain, fever and abdominal cramps
botulism	*Clostridium botulinum*, an anaerobic, Gram-positive, rod-shaped bacterium	*Clostridium botulinum* produces extremely potent toxins which cause muscle paralysis, progressive muscle weakness, respiratory failure and death; the toxins are destroyed by heating at 80 °C for 30 minutes
typhoid fever	*Salmonella typhi*, a Gram-negative, rod-shaped bacterium	Initially a flu-like illness, with fever, aches and respiratory symptoms. There may be either diarrhoea or constipation. If untreated, the fever increases and 'rose spots' may appear on the skin of the upper abdomen. Before antibiotics were available, 12 to 16% of patients died
polio	Poliovirus, an example of an enterovirus, which contains RNA	Poliovirus invades the central nervous system after ingestion of contaminated food or water. Symptoms include fever and sore throat, followed by muscle paralysis
cholera	*Vibrio cholerae*, a Gram-negative, comma-shaped bacterium	*Vibrio cholerae* produces a toxin which causes severe, watery diarrhoea, known as 'rice water stool' because of its appearance. Considerable fluid loss results in severe dehydration; if untreated, cholera has a mortality rate of 40 to 60%

Figure 2.8 shows the number of reported cases of food poisoning in England and Wales during 1987. Describe how the incidence of food poisoning varies during the year and suggest reasons for the variations you have described. What are the implications for the control of food poisoning?

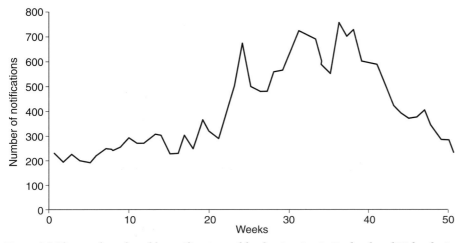

Figure 2.8 The number of weekly notifications of food poisoning in England and Wales during 1987

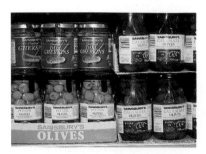

Figure 3.1 Olives and gherkins – some preserved foods which have now become speciality or gourmet foods

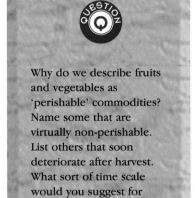

Why do we describe fruits and vegetables as 'perishable' commodities? Name some that are virtually non-perishable. List others that soon deteriorate after harvest. What sort of time scale would you suggest for some of the products you have listed?

Postharvest changes

When you pick an apple off a tree, it does not die – living metabolic processes continue for days, weeks or even months afterwards. Internal physiological changes occur which affect its chemical composition, colour, taste, texture and mass. Some of these changes contribute to qualities associated with ripeness, others lead ultimately to deterioration, spoilage and decay. In the home or in traditional rural communities, a host of strategies has been developed which conserve or preserve fresh food so that it can be eaten at a later date, usually to tide over seasons when food would be scarce or unavailable. Out of this a whole range of specialist foods have developed. These include jams and jellies, dried and crystallised fruits, pickled and fermented vegetables, smoked and pickled fish, smoked and salted meats.

The development of the food industry is largely a consequence of the shift from rural to urban society. In the late 20th century, the food industry is closely linked to the agricultural and horticultural industries with a greater dependence on professional food producers and processors. World-wide trading of perishable goods brings, for example, tropical fruits fresh to the supermarket shelves in the UK, out of season salad crops, unusual vegetables and 'new' potatoes throughout the year.

Substantial losses occur in crops after harvest. Estimates for fresh fruit and vegetables vary between 20 per cent and 80 per cent. Mechanical damage in the form of bruising or splitting can lead to discolouration and changes in flavour. Internal changes, due to enzyme activity, contribute to deterioration and this may be exacerbated by unsuitable storage conditions. Invasion by pathogens may result in fungal or bacterial disease. Attacks by insects, slugs and snails reduce the edible portion of the produce and make it susceptible to microbial decay. On a global scale, post-harvest losses reduce the food available for consumption and this can lead to a serious shortfall in regions where supplies are already inadequate. There are thus strong economic as well as social reasons for understanding the postharvest biology.

In the modern food industry, considerable attention is paid to postharvest conditions for fruit and vegetables, fish and meats, which are destined to be sold fresh, without further processing. The aim of postharvest treatment is to ensure the desired freshness and nutritional value is maintained from the initial handling at harvest or slaughter, then during transport and storage until the produce is presented for sale to the consumer and finally eaten.

Fruits and vegetables

Our fruits and vegetables come from various parts of a plant and are harvested at different stages in the life cycle of the plant. Generally we can recognise three main physiological stages of development, though in the living plant, the boundary between the stages is often indistinct (see Figure 3.2).

- **Growth stage** – cell division and enlargement occur, resulting in rapid increase in size.
- **Physiological maturity** – maximum growth of the plant organ has occurred, often associated with full ripening of a fruit.
- **Senescence** – catabolic processes take over from anabolic processes, leading to degradation rather than synthesis.

Commercial maturity indicates the stage at which the plant organ is ready for the consumer market. This may occur at different developmental stages and does not necessarily coincide with physiological maturity.

For fruits in particular, we talk about **ripeness** as the stage at which it is desirable to eat them. Ripening involves a complex series of physical and biochemical changes and effectively transforms an inedible plant organ into a food that is attractive to eat, from the point of view of its appearance, taste and texture. The flesh of an unripe Conference pear, for example, is hard, gritty, white and with little flavour, but as it ripens it is transformed into a fruit with firm but soft texture, creamy white in colour and dripping with sweet and flavoursome juice. The same pear can soon become mushy and brownish inside, losing its flavour and appeal to the consumer as further changes take place. Courgettes are an example of fruits which are eaten when botanically under-ripe; 'mangetout' peas, French and runner beans, are eaten in their pods, long before the seeds (peas or beans) become mature.

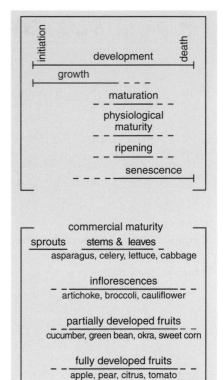

Figure 3.2 Generalised development stages of plants and the stage at which commercial maturity occurs in different fruits and vegetables

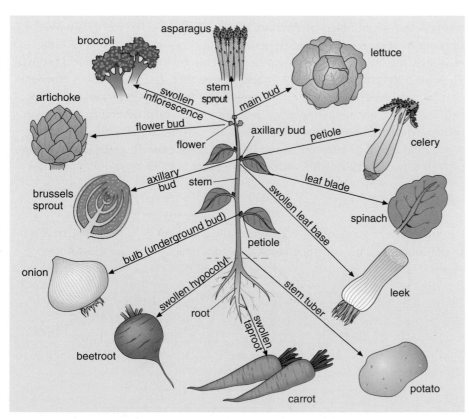

Figure 3.3 Some vegetables and their derivation from different parts of plants

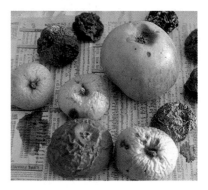

Figure 3.4 Home-grown apples, kept for several months, The apples were stored between layers of newspaper but otherwise had no special treatment

The ripening process

Once picked from the tree, apples can be stored for several months in a cool place without any special treatment. The skin colour changes from green to yellowish or red, the texture softens, the apple becomes sweeter and other subtle changes develop in the flavour. Gradually the apple shrivels, brownish patches become evident and eventually decay sets in.

Table 3.1 *Apple varieties vary in the length of time they keep successfully in storage. All would be kept at 90 to 95% relative humidity*

Apple cultivar	Storage temperature / °C	Storage life / months
Discovery	3.5	1
Worcester Pearmain	0–1.0	2–3
Cox's orange pippin	3.0–3.5	3–4
Bramley's seedling	3.0–4.0	4–5
Tydeman's late orange	3.0–4.0	5
Golden delicious	1.5–2.0	4–6
Granny smith	–1.0–0	3–8

Controlled atmosphere storage is usually 1–2% carbon dioxide and 2–3% oxygen

In an apple, **respiration** continues after it has been harvested. This means that oxygen is taken up, and carbon dioxide, water and heat are given off. Loss of water also occurs by **transpiration**. When the apple is attached to the plant, water and respiratory substrates are replaced from other parts of the plant where active metabolic processes are taking place. Once it has been harvested, the fruit or vegetable becomes dependent upon its own food reserves and moisture. As these are lost they cannot be replaced and deterioration sets in. The rate of respiration (Figure 3.5), goes through a series of changes from the time of petal fall through the development of the fruit. The increased rate of respiration accompanying ripening is known as the **climacteric**, a feature shown in some fruits and vegetables. Linked with the climacteric peak in respiration rate is an increase in the production of **ethene (ethylene)**, a plant growth substance associated with the processes of ripening.

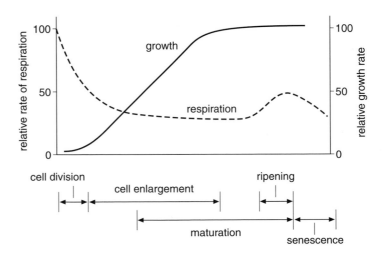

Figure 3.5 Changes in respiration rate in apples or pears from early development of the fruit through the stages of ripening and senescence

After an apple has been picked, various physiological changes associated with ripening and senescence become evident.:

- **Pectic substances** in the middle lamella break down, giving softer texture in the fruit.
- **Chlorophyll** is degraded, leading to loss of the green colour. Yellows and reds of carotenoids, anthocyanins and other pigments become visible in a ripe apple.
- **Organic acid** levels fall, accompanied by increased sugar content. The balance between sugars and acids makes an important contribution to taste, in terms of sweetness or sourness. In apples, malic acid is the main organic acid found and some is used as a respiratory substrate. Sugars include fructose, glucose and sucrose.
- **Volatile substances** present in minute quantities contribute to the characteristic flavours. In green apples the compound 2-hexenel is an important component of the aroma, whereas in ripe apples ethyl 2-methylbutyrate is present. Other flavour and aroma compounds are synthesised during ripening.

Botanically the tomato is a fruit, even though it is classed as a vegetable for eating. Like the apple, respiration and other metabolic activities continue in the tomato up to and beyond the stage of ripeness and harvest. Starch tends to accumulate before ripeness, to be replaced by fructose and glucose as the tomato ripens, giving the characteristic sweetness of ripe tomatoes. Cherry tomatoes are notable because they contain some sucrose. These sugars account for about 65 per cent of the total 'soluble solids' in tomatoes. Malic, citric and ascorbic acids are among those which contribute to the sourness or acidity and, as the tomato ripens, the acidity decreases and sweetness increases. In addition, there are around 400 volatile compounds, present in minute concentrations, which contribute to aroma or flavour. If tomatoes are picked before they are ripe, they have not developed their full sugar content nor do they have the full range of odour compounds. Similarly, if under-ripe tomatoes are kept and refrigerated for a week or so before being eaten, the full potential flavour is not reached. The colours in tomatoes are due to carotenoid pigments – carotenes show as orange and lycopene gives the red. These pigments are significant in that their development is associated with other metabolic changes and so are useful as indicators of the stage of ripeness (see Figure 3.7).

Ethene has a very important role in ripening of fruits. It is often referred to as ethylene in the commercial world and by research workers involved with fruits and vegetables. Ethene is a gas, and is synthesised from the amino acid methionine through a series of intermediates, including a compound abbreviated as ACC. An increase in ethene is associated with the rise in respiration before the onset of ripening. Ethene has an important role in the switching on and off of genes involved in the ripening programme, by activating genes controlling colour, texture and flavour (Figure 3.6). Of particular interest is the production of ethene and the relationship between polygalacturonase and firmness (see Figure 3.7). Pectinesterase (PE) and polygalacturonase (PG) are two enzymes involved in the stages of breakdown of pectic substances in the cell wall, through the pathway

$$\text{propectin} \rightarrow \text{pectinic acid} \xrightarrow{\text{PE}} \text{pectic acid} \xrightarrow{\text{PG}} \text{galacturonic acid}$$

In pears, using the Conference cultivar, measurements of the starch content can be used as an indicator of its stage of ripeness. The cut surface of a pear is dipped into a solution containing 4 per cent potassium iodide and 1 per cent iodine. Harvesting is carried out when the cut surface shows 65–70 per cent blue black. When eating fruit, how do you judge its ripeness? Think about taste in relation to sugar content and acidity. How far does colour influence your perception of acceptability of the fruit?

Breakdown of the pectic substances is largely responsible for the changes in texture leading to mushiness in the overripe tomato or to the softer texture in apples when they are kept over a period of time. The enzyme PG is absent, or present in only very low quantities in unripe fruit, but is found in large quantities in ripe fruit. It acts by reducing the chain length of pectin molecules in the middle lamella and primary cell wall (see Chapter 4). Similarly, in apples the softening of the fruit is due to degradation of pectic substances in the cell wall.

Figure 3.6 Ethene has a key role in switching on and off the genes involved in the ripening process

Look at Table 3.2 and Figure 3.8 which summarise changes in a banana fruit during ripening.
What is used as a measure of respiration? Is this a climacteric fruit, like the apple? Suggest why the transpiration rate goes up sharply in the later stages.
Why does the dry matter decrease? What do you think will be happening to the overall loss in mass?
What makes ripe bananas much sweeter than unripe ones?
What other differences do you notice when eating a *very* unripe banana, a ripe one and an overripe one?

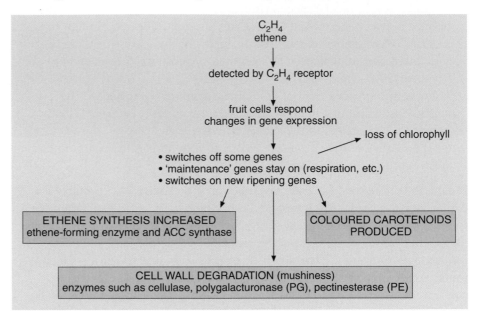

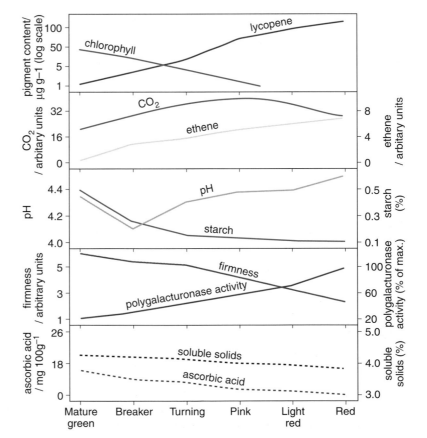

Figure 3.7 Some changes that occur during the ripening of tomato fruit

Table 3.2 *Colour stages and changes in starch–sugar balance in ripening bananas*

Stage	Colour of peel	Approx. starch (%)	Approx. sugar (%)	Comments
1	green	20	0.5	hard, rigid; no ripening
sprung	green	19.5	1.0	bends slightly, ripening started
2	green, trace of yellow	18	2.5	
3	more green than yellow	16	4.5	
4	more yellow than green	13	7.5	
5	yellow, green tip	7	13.5	
6	full yellow	2.5	18	peels readily; firm ripe
7	yellow, lightly flecked with brown	1.5	19	fully ripe; aromatic
8	yellow with increasing brown areas	1.0	19	overripe; pulp soft and darkening, highly aromatic

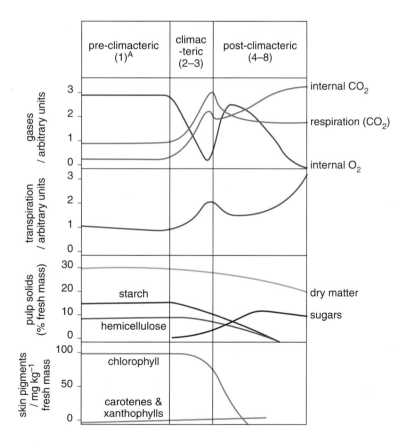

Figure 3.8 Summary of some biochemical changes in banana fruit during ripening. Actual values of gas concentrations and transpiration vary considerably in different conditions and the curves for overripe fruit are very variable. The numbers refer to stages given in Table 3.2

Some postharvest changes in fruits of the cucurbit family:

- Cucumbers, when freshly picked, are green and sometimes slightly bitter in taste. When kept with no special treatment for several weeks after harvest, they become yellow, quite soft and juicy and fairly sweet.
- Overgrown courgettes grow into marrows, which can be stored for several months after harvest without special treatment. Their flesh turns orange in colour and their outer skin becomes quite hard.

Why do you think cucumbers are often offered for sale wrapped in a thin polythene sleeve?

What changes might be taking place in the flesh of the mature marrow? How could you find out if the marrow becomes sweeter? Describe how you could monitor changes in the sweetness of the cucumber and the marrow – qualitatively and quantitatively.

Do you think you could use mature marrow flesh as a substitute for pumpkin to make a sweet pumpkin pie?

How does the outer skin of the mature marrow help to give it an extended storage life?

Meat

Meat is derived from the muscle of an animal. It is made up of bundles of microscopic fibres, with associated connective tissue and fat around and between the bundles. A young animal has a higher proportion of bone in its body weight and a mature animal has a greater deposition of fat. The breed can affect both the distribution of muscle and the rate at which growth occurs. The quality of the meat depends on a number of factors, including the breed of the animal, the feeding strategy used, its sex, age at slaughter and the treatment immediately before and after slaughter.

Up to the moment of slaughter, the muscle has been carrying out metabolic processes, notably respiration. When the animal is killed, a series of irreversible biochemical changes occur, which affect the eating quality of meat and, if not controlled, would lead to deterioration and finally spoilage. In the living animal, contraction of muscle involves the proteins **actin** and **myosin**. The process requires a supply of energy released from ATP, which is replenished from glycogen reserves in the muscle. Energy is also required to maintain the temperature and organisation of the cells. At the moment of death, blood circulation ceases as does the supply of oxygen to the muscle. At first glycogen continues to be broken down and glycolysis results in the anaerobic production of lactate (lactic acid). Accumulation of lactate causes a fall in pH, leading to inactivation of the enzymes involved in ATP release. In the absence of ATP, actin and myosin combine to form rigid chains of actomyosin. The muscle contracts but is unable to relax again. This condition is known as *rigor mortis*. Before rigor mortis, the meat is always tender, but if the muscle is cooked while in the state of rigor mortis, the meat is tougher and darker in colour than it would be if cooked before the condition sets in or after it has passed through rigor. In the present day systems of commercial distribution, meat is not available to the consumer until after rigor.

After rigor mortis, the muscle goes through a period of **ageing**, also known as **conditioning**. Ageing allows development of flavour and the meat becomes more tender. Changes occur in the proteins of the muscle resulting in their becoming more pliable, hence more tender on cooking. This is accompanied by some enzymatic breakdown of protein into peptides and amino acids. To reduce the chance of microbial infection, the meat is kept at temperatures around 5 °C and in clean conditions. Meat may be hung for up to two weeks or longer, depending on the age of the meat and conditions under which it is kept.

The level of glycogen in the muscle before slaughter is a critical factor in developing the desired quality in meat. As glycogen is converted into lactate, the pH of the meat falls, from about 7.4 to 5.5. This helps to improve its texture and keeping qualities. If the pH is too high, the meat is likely to have poor colour with a reduced water-holding capacity. The meat is more susceptible to attack by microorganisms and does not keep well. Pre-slaughter treatment can directly affect glycogen levels. Any form of stress, perhaps during the loading and unloading of animals for transport, fighting, struggling or other exercise leads to depletion of glycogen reserves. Similarly, poor nutrition of the animal, particularly in the period before slaughter, results in low glycogen levels. Pigs are more sensitive than cattle to depletion of glycogen and in some cases the animals are rested after transport or fed with sugar before killing to allow replenishment of glycogen reserves.

Tenderisation of meat can be hastened by the use of **protease** enzymes. The practice is not new and was probably carried out at least 500 years ago by Mexican Indians who wrapped meat in pawpaw leaves during cooking. An enzyme known as **papain**, extracted from the latex of the pawpaw plant (*Carica papaya*) is now the most widely used proteolytic enzyme and shows activity with actomyosin, collagen and elastin. Other proteases used include **ficin** from the fig plant, **bromelin** from the pineapple and some of bacterial and fungal origin. These enzymes can be administered by injection, shortly before slaughter. They appear to have little or no effect on the live animal because the pH of the blood is well above their optimum and the *in vivo* oxygen tensions are unsuitable. The enzymes reach their optimum temperature for activity at about 70 to 85 °C, temperatures which are achieved during cooking. This treatment reduces the time needed for post-slaughter storage. Treatments such as salt and marinating with wine or vinegar also act as tenderisers of meat proteins.

Colour plays an important part in the marketing of meat. To the consumer, good eating quality and freshness are associated with a red colour in meat. The red colour is due primarily to the **myoglobin** in the muscle, rather than haemoglobin of the blood. The actual colour of the meat surface depends on the type of myoglobin molecule and also on its chemical state. The myoglobin molecule consists of one haem unit joined to one protein molecule. It is the iron within the haem unit which is the key to the colour changes (Figure 3.10). The bright red colour on the surface of meat is due mainly to **oxymyoglobin**.

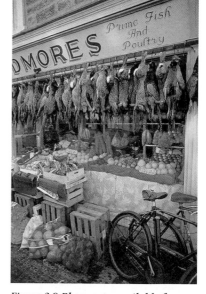

Figure 3.9 Pheasants available for sale. Hanging meat after slaughter makes it more tender and allows certain flavours to develop

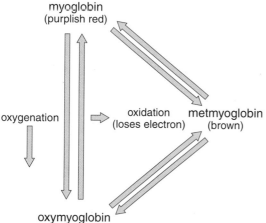

- **myoglobin**, iron (II), purplish-red colour
- **oxymyoglobin**, iron (II), formed from myoglobin by **oxygenation** - molecule of oxygen binds onto the haem unit, bright red colour
- **metmyoglobin**, iron (III), formed from myoglobin or oxymyoglobin by **oxidation** - iron (II) loses and electron to become iron (III), brown colour

The reactions are reversible, so myoglobin is formed by reduction of metmyoglobin or de-oxygenation of oxymyoglobin. The bright red colour on the surface of meat is due mainly to oxymyoglobin. The dull brown sometimes seen on the lower side of fresh meat standing on a container, results from development of metmyoglobin, due to lack of oxygen. The brown colour of cooked meat is due to denatured myoglobin.

- **nitrosomyoglobin** is the bright pink colour of cured meat, formed by the combination of myoglobin with nitric oxide used in the curing process

Figure 3.10 Changes in myglobin in relation to colour in meat

Short and long term storage

In primitive communities, the ability to store harvested crops even for short periods was an important step in the development of agriculture. In the modern food industry, the storage system used is determined by the nature of

FOOD STORAGE

How would you define spoilage? What do you associate with food that is spoiled, that makes it unpleasant or unfit for consumption? Think about texture, colour, taste and odour, then see how far these fit your perception of spoiled food:

• sour milk and yoghurt or other fermented milk
• putrefying chicken and game hung to 'mature'.

the food product and linked closely to marketing strategies. Short-term storage may just be temporary, as in the collection of harvested produce to allow enough to accumulate to send on to market, or it may be appropriate for some crops intended for local use or for consumption in a matter of days or a few weeks after harvest – highly perishable fruits and vegetables, such as strawberries or lettuces, have a limited life. Longer term storage may extend over a period of weeks, months or even years. Produce that is stored over longer periods can then be transported and distributed over considerable distances, even globally.

Our review of post-harvest changes indicates that fruits and vegetables deteriorate for a number of reasons:

• loss of water, leading to limpness or shrivelling
• loss of stored respiratory substrate (usually carbohydrate)
• loss of other nutrients, such as vitamins
• changes in taste, because of alteration of the organic acid and sugar balance
• other internal enzymatic activities, including development of different aroma compounds
• softening of tissues due to degradation of pectic substances (polygalacturonase and pectic enzyme)
• loss in quality because of other metabolic changes or physiological disorders (such as brown, mealy flesh in apples, or 'bitter pit' which is related to calcium deficiency in apples)
• other changes, such as development of woody fibres, root or shoot growth, germination of seeds or sprouting (e.g. onions, potatoes)

Browning occurs as a result of enzyme action. Polyphenol oxidases (phenolases) act on phenolic compounds, such as catechol in apples, converting them to dark-coloured compounds in the group known as tannins. This oxidative browning is commonly seen on the cut surface of fruits such as apples or avocados when exposed to air. Browning can also occur as a result of injury from chilling or bruising.

Suggest why there is less browning when potatoes are peeled under water which has been boiled then cooled, or why lemon juice is squeezed on to sliced avocados and bananas.

As well as these internal changes, there may be physical losses through **pests** or **disease** and saprophytic attack by **microorganisms**. A wide range of microorganisms is likely to be on the surface of any harvested fruits or vegetables. Others may be introduced during processing. Microorganisms are very diverse, but for growth they must have moisture, a suitable temperature together with a source of energy (usually carbohydrate), plus nitrogen and other nutrients. Many require oxygen but some are anaerobic. Their growth is likely to be sensitive to pH – bacteria are less tolerant of acid conditions than yeasts or moulds. Any food destined for humans is probably also a suitable environment for microorganisms, whose metabolic activities are then liable to alter the composition and texture of the food, often making it unfit for human consumption. Bacteria are less likely to grow on fruits because of their high sugar content, but moulds soon grow on the sugary juices, particularly if there is any damage to the skin surface.

In addition to the post-slaughter changes which take place within meat, spoilage may occur as a result of infecting organisms, which may either be present in the living animal or acquired through contamination during the post-slaughter period. Examples of internal infecting organisms include the bacteria *Bacillus anthracis* which causes anthrax, *Mycobacterium tuberculosis* which causes tuberculosis and various species of the genus *Salmonella*, which cause food poisoning (see Chapter 2). Meats may also be infected with parasitic worms, such as the beef tapeworm (*Taenia saginata*) or a variety of nematode worms. Regulations regarding conditions under which the animals are reared as well as inspection of meat at the time of slaughter aim to minimise or detect infected meat.

Spoilage by infection after slaughter, of fresh and refrigerated meats, is mainly from bacteria and moulds, and sometimes yeasts. The contamination may come from hides, hooves or hair and also during the handling and cutting of the meat if this is not done under clean conditions. Microbes growing on the surface are seen as a slimy film. As the microorganisms use the available oxygen, the surface layer may turn brownish due to formation of methaemoglobin. Breakdown of proteins occurs and gases produced include carbon dioxide, hydrogen and ammonia. Later stages of putrefaction are characterised by foul-smelling gases, such as hydrogen sulphide and amines. Growth of contaminating microorganisms is reduced by storage at chill temperatures, usually between 0 and 5 °C. The pH is also important in reducing microbial growth. The production of lactic acid and low pH developed during the conditioning stages are unfavourable for microbial growth.

Table 3.3 *Some symptoms of microbial spoilage of meat*

Type of microorganism	Oxygen status	Spoilage symptoms
bacteria	present	• slime on surface • discolouration (destruction of meat pigments, growth of coloured colonies) • production of gas • off-odours and taints • decomposition of fats
yeasts	present	• slime • discolouration • off-odours and tastes • decomposition of fats
moulds	present	• surface stickiness and whiskers • discolouration • odours and taints • decomposition of fats
bacteria	absent	• putrefaction accompanied by foul odours • production of gases • souring

Storage of fruits and vegetables

The main emphasis of postharvest treatment and conditions used during storage and transport is to:
- minimise water loss
- reduce respiration
- delay ripeness until required by the consumer
- slow the onset of senescence
- avoid spoilage by microorganisms.

Humidity and water loss

Water loss, due to transpiration, can be controlled by increasing the humidity of the storage chamber. This can be achieved by spraying water as a fine mist inside the store. Though the higher humidity favours growth of microorganisms, many fresh fruits and vegetables are stored in a relative humidity between 85 and 95 per cent. Damage to the skin surface is liable to increase the rate of water loss. The natural surface of fruits and some vegetables is often waxy and can play a part in minimising water loss. To help reduce weight loss, artificial waxes have been developed which are applied as a film on the outside of fruits such as apples, citrus fruits and avocado pears. Fungicides and inhibitors of senescence can be incorporated into the wax formulation. Such coatings also affect the gas exchange, by allowing oxygen to diffuse into the apple but retaining some of the carbon dioxide produced in respiration. This effectively modifies the internal atmosphere, which also prolongs the life of the stored apple. Sometimes fruit with these coatings is polished, to increase the sales appeal. The wrapping and packaging also affect the humidity immediately around the fruit or vegetable. Leafy vegetables, such as lettuce or spinach, soon wilt unless moisture can be retained within suitable packaging.

Temperature

Most fruits and vegetables are stored at temperatures lower than their growing environment; some are pre-cooled at the time of harvest. Tomatoes are often cooled after picking by being tipped into a bath of cold water at 10 °C. Lettuces may be chilled by 'vacuum cooling'. For this, they are placed in boxes in a vacuum chamber and some moisture is boiled off. Alternatively, lettuces may be packed for transport in boxes surrounded with ice. Low temperatures reduce the rate of respiration hence the disappearance of respiratory substrate. A temperature between 1 °C and 4 °C is suitable for storing apples, and this also diminishes attack by fungi and bacteria. Below 0 °C, the tissues may suffer from irreversible chilling injury, since frozen tissues may fail to resume metabolic processes when thawed. This can result in permanent browning and damage. The critical temperature for chilling injury varies with different cultivars and different crops. Potatoes should not be stored below a temperature of 4 °C because this favours conversion of starch to sugars. Lowering the temperature decreases the rate of ethene production and the response of tissues to the effects of ethene, thus delaying the onset of ripening. The development of the aroma in ripe fruit and the green colour turning to yellow, are also slower at lower temperatures. The actual temperature inside the fruit or vegetable, is likely to be higher than that set for the storage chamber due to the heat generated in respiration. The store should provide continual cooling, if necessary by air circulation with fans, to ensure the desired temperature is maintained. However, air circulation will encourage loss of water, so a balance must be found.

Storage atmosphere

Modification of the gases in the atmosphere in which apples are stored has led to considerable success in prolonging the storage life. The terms **controlled atmosphere** (CA) or **modified atmosphere** (MA), are used to describe

QUESTION

In **controlled atmosphere** storage systems, the gas composition is carefully monitored and actively controlled. In **modified atmosphere** storage systems, the produce is held in an airtight store and the respiration of the produce is allowed to change the composition of the atmosphere.

systems in which the atmospheric composition is different from normal air. The practice has ancient origins: burying of apples or carrying them in unventilated holds of ships resulted in a much longer storage life. The effect was probably due to lower oxygen and higher carbon dioxide in the surrounding atmosphere, modified as a result of respiration in the tissue.

In modern storage systems, the atmosphere is deliberately manipulated, with levels of oxygen, carbon dioxide, nitrogen, ethylene and carbon monoxide being controlled. Storage containers must be sealed and monitored closely. Respiration of the stored produce leads to a fall in oxygen concentration and rise in carbon dioxide concentration. In some cases nitrogen gas is introduced to ensure the crop rapidly reaches the required levels of oxygen and carbon dioxide. Because respiration continues, fresh air is introduced to maintain the required level of oxygen. Carbon dioxide is produced from the stored product and chemical absorbants are used to prevent the level getting too high. Controlled atmosphere storage has been applied mainly to stored apples, but it is being used increasingly with other crops, including bananas, avocados, tomatoes, cucumbers, Chinese cabbage, broccoli and potatoes.

In apples stored at 5 °C, the oxygen level must be reduced to 2.5 per cent to achieve a 50 per cent reduction in respiration. Care must be taken to ensure conditions do not become anaerobic as this could lead to development of undesirable flavours. At higher temperatures with low oxygen, anaerobic respiration increases. Increased carbon dioxide levels also affect respiration: for apples, a storage atmosphere with carbon dioxide levels between 5 per cent and 10 per cent is often used but if higher, anaerobic respiration can occur. Low oxygen and high carbon dioxide both delay ripening and the breakdown of chlorophyll, and also reduce ethene production. This atmosphere also reduces the breakdown of pectic substances in the middle lamella, keeping the texture firm for longer. With prolonged storage in low oxygen and high carbon dioxide undesirable flavours and odours may develop. High levels of carbon dioxide also reduce microbial activity, thus delaying the onset of decay. In practice, different products vary considerably in their tolerance to reduced oxygen and increased carbon dioxide levels, as shown in Table 3.5. Lettuces and other salad crops can, for example, be stored for 4 weeks in containers with an atmosphere of 10 per cent carbon dioxide, 10 per cent oxygen and 80 per cent nitrogen.

Within the storage atmosphere, accumulated ethene encourages the onset of ripening so there should be adequate ventilation inside the storage chamber to remove ethene. Fruits at different stages of ripeness should not be stored together, since ethene produced from riper fruits would affect the less ripe. Chemicals, such as potassium permanganate, can be used to absorb ethene, both in the incoming air and inside the container itself. Bunches of bananas are sometimes sealed inside polyethylene bags, on or off the plant, to delay the ripening process. This is a relatively simple way for the subsistence farmer to create a modified atmosphere on the farm, though ethene tends to accumulate (Table 3.4).

Table 3.4 *Bananas and storage life – effect of sealing in polyethylene bags and use of potassium permanganate. Inclusion of potassium permanganate can result in the shelf life being noticeably extended*

Treatment (bananas)	Shelf life / days
air control	up to 7
sealed polyethylene bags	14
sealed bags + potassium permanganate	21

Table 3.5 *Recommended storage conditions for a selection of fruits and vegetables.*

Fruit or vegetable	Temperature / °C	RH (%)	Storage life	Controlled atmosphere (CA) effects
banana	11–14	85–90	2–3 weeks	5% Co_2, 4% O_2, extends shelf life ×3
beetroot	0–4	~95	3–5 months	CA has little effect
broccoli	0	95–100	10–14 days	5–10% CO_2, 1–2% O_2
cabbage	0–2	95	2–6 months	2.5–5% CO_2, 2.5–5% O_2
capsicum (peppers)	7–10	85–95	2–5 weeks	2% CO_2, 4% O_2
carrot	0	95	4–8 months	CA not recmmended
cauliflower	0–1	85–95	2–6 weeks	CA has liitle effect
courgette	5–10	90–95	2–3 weeks	CA has little effect
cucumber	7–10	85–95	1–2 weeks	5–7% CO_2, 3–5% O_2
lemon	8–12	85–90	1–3 months	5–10% CO_2, 5% O_2
lettuce	0	90–95	1–3 weeks	1.5%$_2$, 3% O_2
mango	7–13	85–90	2–7 weeks	5% CO_2, 5% O_2
marrow	10–15	70–75	2–6 months	CA has little effect
mushroom	0	95	3–10 days	10–15% CO_2, 21% O_2
onion	0	65–75	6–8 months	CA has variable success
parsnip	0	90–95	2–6 months	quality and sweetness improve after exposure to frost
peas (mangetout)	0	90–95	1–2 weeks	5–7% CO_2, 5–10% O_2
potatoes	7–10	85–95	4–8 months	CA has variable effects. Below 4°C potatoes become sweeter
raspberries	0	85–95	3–7 days	CA has little effect

Storage life depends on a combination of temperature, humidity and gas atmosphere. Values given in the table are representative of a range, which can vary considerably with different varieties of fruits and vegetables, and sometimes recommendations extend outside the ranges given. For some crops, such as beetroot, courgettes and cauliflower, modified atmospheres appear to give no improvement in storage life. Where CA is not recommended, it may be that decay or spoilage increases with the controlled atmosphere.

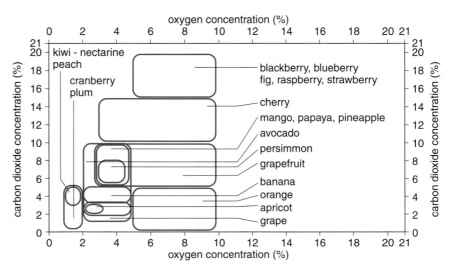

Figure 3.11 Recommended modified atmospheres for storage of a selection of fruits

Storage of meats

The factors affecting storage of fresh and cut meat are similar to those described for fruits and vegetables. Unprotected meat readily loses **water** by evaporation with a consequent loss in weight and deterioration in appearance. processes, some of which are beneficial. For short-term storage, meat is usually kept between 0 and 4 °C to minimise microbial spoilage, though certain microorganisms do grow at these temperatures. The composition of the **gases** around the surface of the meat is important both for the colour of the meat surface and in determining the extent of microbial growth. **Oxygen** is required to maintain the bright red colour of meat. The actual composition of the atmosphere is one factor that determines the species of microorganism which grow on the meat – some are favoured by aerobic conditions whereas others can grow only in anaerobic conditions. Changes in colour or development of undesirable odours as a result of bacterial or mould growth, are often evident before other signs of spoilage. True putrefaction with development of foul-smelling compounds is due to the decomposition of proteins in anaerobic conditions, usually by *Clostridium* spp. High **carbon dioxide** concentrations tend to have an inhibitory effect on the growth of certain microorganisms. As with fruit and vegetables, manipulation of the atmospheric gases can make a useful contribution to prolonging the storage life of cut meat.

Preservation of foods

Preservation of food implies treatment in ways that will protect the food from spoilage by microorganisms, deterioration as a result of enzyme activity or by oxidation. Methods used for preservation often bring about changes in the physical nature and taste of foods. The main emphasis is to reduce microbial decay rather than maintain the same qualities as in fresh food. Storage of foods preserved by freezing, canning and dehydration is expected to be fairly long term, probably months or years, rather than days or weeks. Food can, of course, be frozen one day and thawed for consumption the next.

Short-term treatments keep the food fit for consumption for days or weeks rather than months. **Blanching** and **cooking** can be thought of as short-term methods of preservation. When blanching, the food is plunged into hot water for up to 5 minutes. This inactivates enzymes which would lead to internal breakdown of cells and tissues, known as autolysis. During cooking, temperatures inside foods may reach about 70 °C and this destroys most, but not necessarily all, of the microorganisms in or around the food. **Refrigeration**, or **chilling**, is useful for the short-term preservation of many foods. Refrigerators are usually maintained at temperatures between 1 and 4 °C, since most pathogenic bacteria are unable to multiply below 4 °C.

Raw food materials for freezing, canning and dehydration are cleaned, sorted on the basis of size, shape, colour or other features and graded on the basis of quality. Fruits and vegetables are usually blanched. Most foods are frozen from the raw state, but some foods for canning are pre-cooked.

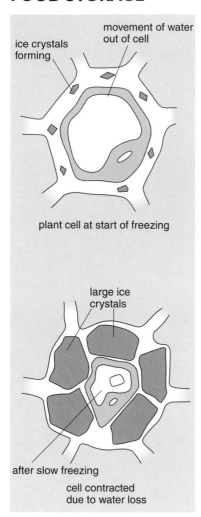

ice crystals forming

movement of water out of cell

plant cell at start of freezing

large ice crystals

after slow freezing

cell contracted due to water loss

Figure 3.12 Plant cells and the formation of ice crystals on freezing

Freezing

Stored frozen foods are generally held at a temperature of about –20 °C, though sometimes temperatures as low as –80 °C are used. The low temperature inhibits microbial growth and may cause death of some microorganisms. Activity of enzymes, and most chemical reactions, is severely retarded. The production of ice within the cells draws out water, so the tissues effectively become dehydrated which further reduces the likelihood of microbial growth. After freezing and thawing, many fruits and vegetables are noticeably altered in texture and sometimes taste though other foods, including meats and fish, compare well with the fresh condition. Freezing is now used widely, both commercially and in the home, for storage of freshly harvested foods, during their transport then in the home for convenience until required for eating.

Plant tissues (fruits and vegetables) when prepared for freezing are often blanched. This lessens the degradation of desirable nutrients or other components, reduces the microorganisms associated with the food and also displaces air trapped within the tissues. In some vegetables, blanching has the advantage of enhancing the green colour (e.g. peas, broccoli). During the freezing process, ice crystals form and water is drawn out of the cells. This makes the remaining solution of salts, sugars and organic acids more concentrated and thus depresses the freezing point (think about salt on icy roads in winter). The temperature inside the tissue may have to fall to about –5 °C or lower before the water in the tissue is really frozen. If the freezing is done slowly, large ice crystals tend to form outside plant cells and, on thawing, the cells will have lost their turgor and liquid (juice) flows quite freely. Quick freezing methods aim to reduce this effect, because the ice crystals which form while the water is still inside the cells are smaller. This means less physical damage inside the tissue due to the ice crystals and the texture remains more like that of the original produce.

Canning

Canning is a form of heat sterilisation. The food is placed in a sealed can or other container and heated to a high temperature with the aim of killing all microorganisms. Traditionally, canning has been done in tins or glass containers, but now trays and pouches made of heat-resistant laminates of polymer materials and foil are being used. These are referred to as 'hermetically sealed containers'. Some bacterial spores do survive the heat treatment. If a can is 'blown' it is a sign that bacterial activity has resumed and such cans must be discarded. Of particular concern is the bacterium *Clostridium botulinum*, which can live in anaerobic conditions and even at low pH its spores can survive some heat treatments. The toxins produced by *C. botulinum* cause food poisoning known as **botulism**.

Fruits and vegetables may be blanched before canning. This also helps to soften them so that they can be packed into the container. Some foods are cooked before being canned. The container must be filled to ensure the contents are immersed in liquid. Sometimes this is done under low pressure before the lid is finally sealed. Sterilisation is carried out at temperatures of 100 °C or above (usually 115 °C or higher for meats and vegetables). The food is heated in sealed containers in steam under pressure. It is the temperature inside the food that is critical in ensuring successful sterilisation. The time for which the food is held at that temperature during the canning process depends on the type of food, its pH and the size of the container being used. Sugary foods and those with low pH need less heating, because of the osmotic effects or intolerance of microorganisms to acid conditions. The size of the container and nature of the food helps determine the heat penetration throughout the container, and the effectiveness of sterilisation. After heating, the can is immediately cooled in cold water. Flaws in the container at this stage could allow entry of microorganisms if the water is contaminated. Canned food invariably differs in texture and taste from the original food, but keeping times are long, provided the canning processing was carried out successfully.

Pasteurised and sterilised milk

Treatment of milk by pasteurisation or sterilisation illustrates the effects of different heat treatments and the distinction between short-term and long term storage. In the UK, about 93 per cent of milk is pasteurised, and the rest is either ultra heat treated (UHT) or sterilised. Only a fraction is sold as unpasteurised milk. Pasteurised milk is popular because the flavour and nutritional content is hardly affected by the pasteurisation process. Pasteurisation aims to kill pathogenic organisms and to reduce the number of other non-pathogenic bacteria which would cause spoilage. Pasteurisation is not effective against spores. In particular, pasteurisation is expected to make the milk safe from *Mycobacterium tuberculosis*, and from *Brucella abortus*, the causative organisms of tuberculosis and brucellosis respectively. Pasteurisation extends the keeping time of the milk for a few days, provided it is kept refrigerated (between 1 and 4 °C). Sterilisation uses heat but at a higher temperature than pasteurisation and aims to destroy bacteria and other microorganisms which may not have been killed by pasteurisation, though some very resistant spores may survive the process.

Pasteurisation is carried out either by heating the milk at a temperature of 62.8 to 65.6 °C for at least 30 minutes, or by heating to 71.7 °C for at least 15 seconds. This 'high-temperature short-time' (HTST) system is now widely used. The milk is passed through pipes or between plates in a heat exchanger system, surrounded by hot water kept at a temperature just above the required temperature. It is carefully controlled to ensure the milk is held at the correct temperature for the appropriate time, then rapidly cooled to about 3 °C. The effectiveness of pasteurisation is checked using the **phosphatase test**. The enzyme phosphatase is slightly more resistant to heat than the bacterium *Mycobacterium tuberculosis*, so a test is carried out on the milk to check that the phosphatase in the milk has been inactivated. The chemical compound known as disodium *p*-nitrophenyl phosphate is added. If active phosphatase is present, this chemical breaks down, producing *p*-nitrophenol, which is detected because it gives a yellow colouration.

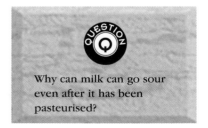

Why can milk can go sour even after it has been pasteurised?

Temperatures used for sterilisation are at least 100 °C, though often the milk is sealed into bottles and heated to a temperature of approximately 115 °C for 20 minutes, then cooled rapidly. The milk can then keep for several months without refrigeration, but the flavour is noticeably altered by the cooking, resulting in a caramelised taste. It has also become homogenised with loss of separated cream. There is some loss of nutrients, compared with raw fresh milk or pasteurised milk. UHT milk (ultra-high-temperature sterilisation) is prepared by heating milk to at least 132.2 °C for at least one second. It is sealed in cartons, aseptically packaged in sterile conditions. UHT milk has a keeping time of several months with flavour qualities close to that of pasteurised milk.

Table 3.6 *Nutrient quality different milks*

Nutrient	Type of milk – composition as g per 100 g				
	Channel islands	Whole	Skimmed	UHT	Sterilised whole
water	86.4	87.8	91.3	87.8	87.8
total fat	4.9	3.9	0.1	3.9	3.9
(of which saturates)	3.1	2.5	0.06	2.5	2.5
protein	3.6	3.2	3.3	3.2	3.2
carbohydrate	4.6	4.6	4.8	4.6	4.6
calcium / mg	131	115	120	115	115
vitamin A / μg	60	53	Trace	53	53
riboflavin / mg	0.19	0.17	0.18	0.17	0.17
vitamin D / μg	0.04	0.03	Trace	0.03	0.03
energy / kJ 100^{-1}	320	276	140	276	276

Dehydration

Drying foods has, for many centuries, been a successful way of preserving fish and meats, fruit and some vegetables. Microbial growth stops when the water content falls below a certain level. Dehydration is similar to freezing in that the microorganisms are not killed, and activity may resume when the available water again reaches a suitable level. The water availability in a food is generally expressed as *water activity* (a_w). Moisture levels are compared with water, which has a water activity of 1.0. Most bacteria cannot grow below an a_w of 0.9, whereas yeasts can tolerate an a_w down to 0.85 and moulds down to about 0.7. Dehydrated foods generally have an aw below 0.6, equivalent to less than 25 per cent of water.

In parts of the world where the sun is hot enough and the atmosphere is dry, dehydration is a simple process. The produce, such as raisins, prunes, dried apricots and pears, is spread on trays in the sun and turned occasionally. Fish and meat can be hung on racks in the air. Otherwise, heated air can be forced over the food. Some dehydrated foods are prepared by freeze drying. The food is frozen, then water is removed by conversion from ice straight to vapour, a process known as sublimation. The quality of freeze-dried food is good but the process is expensive. Dehydrated food is generally soaked in water before being eaten, but rarely recovers its former texture and taste.

Preservation by salting and high sugar concentration effectively lowers the a_w (available water) due to the osmotic effects of the added salt or sugar. Traditional methods of salting and smoking of fish and meat preserve the food mainly through the effect of dehydration. Some modern methods of curing bacon and other fish and meats are less effective for preservation. The treatment is given to modify flavour and simulate the smoking process, but we should still rely on refrigeration for short-term storage to avoid spoilage by microorganisms.

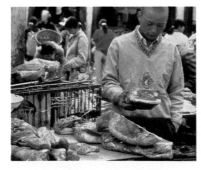

Figure 3.13 Traditional cured hams for sale in a street market in Yunnan, south-west China

Use of chemicals for preservation

Various chemicals are used for preservation of foods. They may create conditions which are unsuitable for microbial growth, or prevent other deterioration within the food material. For example, relatively few microorganisms can grow in a **low pH**, hence the preserving effects of **lactic acid** (see Fermentations, Chapter 4) and of **ethanoic acid** (vinegar) used for pickling. Other additives which contribute to the preservation of food are described in Chapter 2.

Packaging

From very early civilisations, people have used natural materials, such as baskets, pottery vessels, gourds and leather to serve as containers for harvested or stored foods. The last few hundred years has seen the development of glass, paper and metal containers, which remain familiar materials used in packaging today. Much more recently, synthetic materials such as cellulose and polyethylene films, expanded polystyrene and other plastics have been adapted for packaging in the food industry with considerable success.

Packaging plays an increasingly important part in the retailing of foods in the modern food industry. It has a key role in **marketing**, promoting the appeal of the food to the customer and provides a means of **identifying** the product. The packaging also contributes to the maintenance of the desired **quality** of the food. Selection and use of appropriate packaging materials is integrated closely with the postharvest biology of the different foods. The discussion here focuses mainly on the packaging of fresh fruits and vegetables, fish and meats, and we refer mainly to the package as presented to the customer in the supermarket or other retail outlet, rather than the wider range of systems adopted at the time of harvesting, and during storage and transport of the products.

At a simple level, the packaging provides a **container** for the produce, in a discreet weight or volume. The container also acts as a **barrier** and so isolates the material from the environment outside the pack. This barrier can prevent contamination of the packed product from dirt, undesirable chemical substances or from microorganisms. Similarly, the barrier should prevent leakage of materials from the inside, say of juice from fruits or meat, or grease from fatty or oily foods. The package can provide **protection** against mechanical damage, from the time of harvest until the product reaches the home of the purchaser. To illustrate the necessity for this you need think no further than the losses incurred through broken eggs or bruised apples. The package must be strong enough to resist vibration, and damage from being compressed or even dropped, but not so heavy that it adds to costs or handling difficulties. For some foods, it is necessary for the package to protect against the effects of **light**.

A food package can be thought of as a small-scale storage system in which **humidity** and **gas atmosphere** are key features. These factors are also discussed in relation to postharvest biology and storage conditions in general (see pages 48–50). With fresh produce, such as apples and lettuce, the barrier

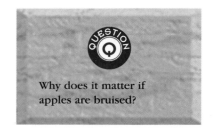

Why does it matter if apples are bruised?

provided by the packaging material can help to reduce water loss by transpiration but it is equally important for the barrier to prevent uptake of water by dry foods, such as dehydrated fruits. However, if the barrier is impermeable to water, with packs of fresh fruits and vegetables, water vapour collects inside the package, and would be evident as condensation or drops of water. In packaged meats, liquid may seep out from exposed surfaces and collect in the container. The pad included inside some packages absorbs this liquid which would otherwise be unsightly. A high relative humidity inside a pack is likely to encourage growth of moulds or other microorganisms which could lead to spoilage. If, however, the barrier is perforated so that it is *partly* permeable, it may still be possible to minimise water loss from the fruit, vegetable or meat but, at the same time, avoid excessive build up of water vapour inside the package.

In a similar way, with plant material, the permeability of the barrier becomes critical with respect to the levels of gases, particularly respiratory gases and **ethene**. If the barrier is impermeable, respiration leads to a depletion of **oxygen** and increase in **carbon dioxide** within the package. While some reduction in oxygen or increase in carbon dioxide slows the postharvest changes associated with ripening and senescence (see pages 38–43), development of anaerobic conditions encourages deterioration of the fruits or vegetables inside the pack. If, however, the pack is *partly* permeable to gases, and perhaps differentially permeable so that the gas composition can be manipulated, we have a powerful tool that can be exploited to control the atmosphere inside the package. This is the basis of **modified atmosphere packaging** (MAP). This technique has been made possible by the development of a range of plastic films, with different permeabilities. Modified atmosphere packaging provides a means of prolonging shelf life of the product as well as being attractive to the consumer in the displays. MAP can be applied to meats and fish as well as to fruits and vegetables and the systems now being used are bringing about a quiet revolution in the food industry.

More questions about apples:
Why does microbial spoilage occur in a pack of apples even if the bag is completely sealed?
What internal changes might take place in apples when the conditions become anaerobic inside the pack?

Table 3.7 *Effects of number and size of perforations in polyethylene bags on storage life of yellow globe onions. The onions were kept in 1.5 kg packs in 150 gauge polyethylene film bags, for 14 days at 24 °C. Measurements were made of the percentage relative humidity inside the bag, the number of onions which rooted and the percentage loss in weight*

Number of perforations	Diameter of perforations / mm	RH in bag (%)	Onions rooted (%)	Loss in mass (%)
0	–	98	71	0.5
36	1.6	88	59	0.7
40	3.2	84	40	1.4
8	6.4	–	24	1.8
16	6.4	54	17	2.5
32	6.4	51	4	2.5

We can distinguish three methods of creating a modified atmosphere (MA) inside the package:

- **passive MA** – in which the high carbon dioxide and low oxygen levels develop passively, as a result of the respiration of the product inside the package. This is relevant particularly with plant material.
- **active MA** – by removing the air originally inside the package and replacing it with the desired gas mixture.
- **active MA with chemicals** – by using chemical substances which will remove or produce the desired changes in the original gas mixture.

Passive MA is probably the least satisfactory, since respiratory activity of fresh produce may vary at different postharvest stages and at different temperatures. With passive MA, it also takes time for the desired gas levels to be achieved. It is more reliable to control the atmosphere by using a vacuum to remove the air from the pack, then flushing it with a gas mixture of the desired composition. Chemical substances which either absorb or generate gases can be placed in sachets inside the package and used to influence the composition of the atmosphere. Examples include powdered ferrous (ironII) compounds, metallic platinum, catechol based compounds and ascorbic acid which act as oxygen 'scavengers'. Ferrous carbonate can be used both to take up oxygen and release carbon dioxide. Potassium permanganate and activated carbon are two substances used to absorb ethene. A further sophistication is to incorporate a colour indicator in the sachet of chemical so that the gas levels inside the packet can be judged, thus giving a measure of the degree of freshness. This is used, for example, in large catering packages but not usually in consumer packages.

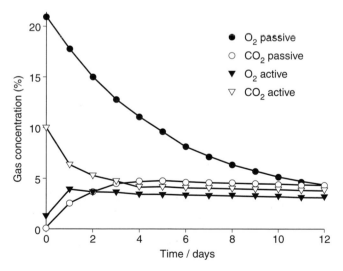

Figure 3.14 Passive compared with active modification – chilli peppers in sealed plastic film packages. Flushing the packages with gases (active modification) brought about a faster change in gas atmosphere

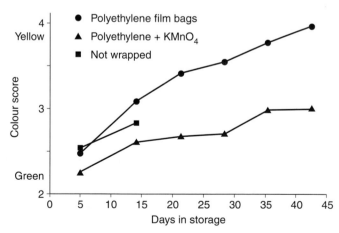

Figure 3.15 Storage of limes and the effects of packaging and of absorbing ethene. The colour score is used as an indicator of ripeness. The limes were kept at 31–34 °C and between 30 and 35% RH

FOOD STORAGE

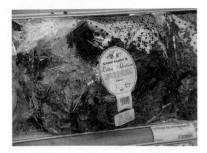

Figure 3.16 Plastic films used for packaging are carefully selected and help prolong the shelf-life of fresh salads

Plantains are tropical fruits which are similar to bananas. Table 3.9 shows how different wrapping materials affected the time to ripeness and weight loss in stored plantains.
• What features could you use to determine the stage of ripeness of the stored plantains?
Suggest why these different packing materials had the effects shown.
For a small-scale farmer, do you think there is any real advantage in wrapping the plantains?
What might be the disadvantages of using polyethylene? Think about costs, labour and the possible environmental consequences as well as the postharvest biology.

With raw meats, the modified atmospheres used may be either high or low in oxygen. The high oxygen MA packs may have up to 80 per cent oxygen, with a balance of either carbon dioxide alone or carbon dioxide with nitrogen. While the presence of oxygen is important for retaining the red colour associated with fresh meat, disadvantages of high oxygen are that it increases the likelihood of rancidity due to oxidation of fats and it is favourable to growth of aerobic microorganisms. The alternative is to have low oxygen, and replace the air with carbon dioxide, or carbon dioxide with nitrogen. This is less suitable for red meats because they discolour to become brownish due to formation of metmyoglobin. The red colour may, however, recover on opening the package and exposure of the contents to oxygen. The high carbon dioxide mixture inhibits growth of a range of microorganisms and does allow considerable increase in shelf life for some meats. In the case of cured meats, oxygen is not required to maintain the pink colour (nitrosomyglobin), so packaging materials for cured meat products should be impermeable to oxygen.

Vacuum packs go a stage further in their control of the atmosphere. The package material must have low permeability to gases, particularly oxygen. This system is now used widely, for example with beef joints packaged immediately after slaughter. The atmosphere around the meat soon becomes low in oxygen and enriched with carbon dioxide. In some cases, as the meat is enclosed in its pack, a vacuum is applied to reduce the gas remaining in the space between the meat and the package film. The oxygen-deficient environment is unsuitable for growth of aerobic microorganisms, provided the pH of the meat is low (less than 5.8). This principle has been exploited with **shrink packs**, used, for example, with frozen poultry. The chicken or meat joint is placed in the bag and a vacuum is applied before sealing. The bag is then heated in warm air or water and the bag shrinks to fit closely around the contours of the meat. A potential danger comes from survival and growth of anaerobic microorganisms inside these packs.

A wide range of plastics are used in packaging in different forms. Development of suitable plastic films has enabled MAP systems to become successful. Four types of film are commonly used: polyvinyl chloride (PVC), polyethylene (PE), polypropylene (PP) and polyethylene terephthalate (PET). There are variations in their properties and selection of the appropriate film requires a number of features to be taken into account:
• **degree of permeability** – to gases (particularly oxygen and carbon dioxide), and to water vapour
• **mechanical** properties – including overall strength, resistance to tearing or bursting under pressure, its ability to be handled by machines, how it can be sealed to form the package or peeled to open the package
• **stability** with respect to **environmental conditions**, particularly changes in temperature and humidity, and ability to withstand conditions during processing such as the high and low temperatures used for sterilisation and freezing
• **visibility** of the product – generally it is more appealing to the consumer to be able to see the fresh produce, though some foods deteriorate more rapidly in the light. This can be counteracted by use of appropriate opaque or dark packaging material, or large labels to cover most of the product.

Care should be taken over possible **interaction** between the packaging material and its contents – that there is no attack on the material from substances in the food and that potentially toxic substances do not migrate from the package to the food.

Table 3.8 *Some packaging films and their permeabilities to gases and to water. Different types of polyvinylchloride (PVC) are given as A, B, C, etc.*

Film type	Thickness / μM	Permeabilities / arbitrary units		
		Oxygen	Carbon dioxide	Water
Polyethylene	12	22 200	96 000	9.3
PVC–A	12	11 000	66 000	300
PVC–B	15	25 000	150 000	110
PVC–C	25	10 000	60 000	70

Finally, we can see how the selection of materials for packaging is linked with the biology of the food material and that the package makes an important contribution to maintaining the freshness of a product. In addition, **labels** on packaged products offer an opportunity for communication with the purchaser, firstly to **identify** the food and then to describe the contents. Increasingly, labelling of food products has a key role in marketing strategies but the information provided must also conform with a range of legislative requirements.

Table 3.9 *Effects of different wrapping and packing materials on ripening and weight loss of plantains, stored at tropical ambient temperatures of between 26 and 34 °C and 52–87% relative humidity*

Packing material	Days to ripeness	Loss in mass at ripeness (%)
not wrapped	15.8	17.0
paper	18.9	17.9
moist coir fibre	27.2	(+3.5)
perforated polyethylene	26.5	7.2
polyethylene	36.1	2.6

Table 3.10 *Changes in nutritional content of 'Satsuma' mandarins after harvest. These mandarins were treated with different edible coatings – 'Semoerfresh' and 'Jonfresh' – then stored at 20 °C and 40% RH. The control had no coating. Changes in ascorbic acid content and in citric acid content were compared over a period of 3 weeks. Coatings provide a modified atmosphere within the fruit, decrease respiration rate, reduce loss of water and can carry fungicides*

Time / weeks	Ascorbic acid / mg 100cm^{-3}			Citric acid (%)		
	Control	Semperfresh	Jonfresh	Control	Semperfresh	Jonfresh
0	25.2	25.2	25.2	1.57	1.57	1.57
1	17.1	18.0	21.1	1.34	1.51	1.50
2	16.6	17.1	20.7	1.06	1.21	1.42
3	14.4	17.1	18.3	0.93	1.25	1.06

QUESTION

Wrapping it all together – the product and the package. Look at a typical range of items for sale in a shop or supermarket. Make a list of the different types of packaging materials used and think of the function each has in relation to the food contained in the package.

• How far does the package influence what you buy? Would you prefer to buy apples, bananas, lettuces, leeks or meat from an open market stall or wrapped in a modified atmosphere package? Try to list reasons for your preference.

• Compare the labels on different sorts of foods. How important to you is the information on the label when you make your selection of foods to buy? What is mandatory to be included on the label? Think whether the other information is useful or why it is presented. Do any of them tell you about the atmosphere inside the pack?

• Some people suggest that packaging must add to the cost of the product and that it is wasteful in terms of resources. How far do you agree with this view? Do you think modern packaging makes a useful contribution to reducing postharvest losses, even on a global scale? What features should be incorporated into packaging materials to minimise environmental impact when the packaging is discarded? How could you help reduce the problem of wastage?

Biotechnology and food production

Biotechnology – ancient and modern

Biotechnology is a relatively modern word, but its roots lie at the very beginnings of human civilisation. The making of bread, cheese and wine are food-processing practices which are central to many human societies, traditional and modern. As humans changed from a hunter-gatherer way of life to more permanent, settled communities, the art of processing food began to develop. The origins of different discoveries were probably accidental, but the benefits were doubtless soon appreciated. Food could be kept longer, transported and stored from one season to the next. A wider range of flavours became part of the diet and alcoholic liquor, particularly, assumed an importance in ceremonies and social gatherings. All this was long before people were aware of the existence of microorganisms, which are the agents responsible for many of these modifications to food.

It was the work of Pasteur in the mid-nineteenth century that led to an understanding of the activities of microorganisms and their role in traditional food processing activities. This signalled the beginnings of microbiology as a science. Today, at the end of the 20th century, biotechnology is concerned with exploiting the activities of living organisms, especially microorganisms. It embraces several disciplines – microbiology, biochemistry and chemistry, cell biology and genetics and engineering to ensure the activities of the organisms can be geared to production, often in large-scale processing. Biotechnology now has medical and agricultural applications, is involved in waste treatment, the production of fuels and in the food and beverage industries. Its future potential is considerable and is likely to increase in the 21st century.

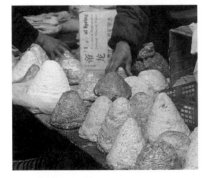

Figure 4.1 Simple cheeses from Yunnan, south-west China, where herds of yaks, cattle, sheep and goats graze the high mountain grassland and the people are essentially pastoralists. The shape of the cheeses is determined by the conical baskets in which the curds drain while the cheese is being made

The ancient art of modifying raw, harvested food has evolved into the modern food processing industry. It is highly mechanised, rigorously monitored and controlled to ensure uniformity of end-products, many of which are destined for world-wide distribution. The impact of biotechnology in the modern food industry can be illustrated by the activities of microorganisms:

- in fermentations
- harvested as biomass to be consumed as food for humans or animals
- in production of extracellular enzymes (see Chapter 2).

In addition, increasingly, we are seeing the application of biotechnology in the formation of products by genetically modified organisms.

Fermentations

The term **fermentation** is used in two senses. In the narrower, biochemical sense, fermentation is a form of **anaerobic respiration**, and is a means by which organisms, or cells within organisms, obtain energy from an organic substrate in the absence of oxygen. In the broader sense, the term is used to describe a very wide range of processes carried out by microorganisms. Many yield products of commercial importance. Some fermentations involve anaerobic respiration, but many do not.

Fermentations are a significant way of modifying raw fresh food. The fermented product has properties that are different from the original plant or animal material. The fermentation may enhance the flavour or alter the texture, palatability and digestibility of the food, and there may be changes in the nutritional content. These changes often make the food safer because it is then unsuitable for the growth of microorganisms and sometimes toxins are eliminated. Traditionally, fermentation of various foods has provided an important means of preservation, though in the modern food industry, other methods, such as freezing, have perhaps become more important.

The fermentations described in this chapter show how different microorganisms are involved and the changes that take place as a result of their metabolism. Often the fermentation leads to a lowering of the pH. This improves the storage properties of the foods because many microorganisms which cause spoilage do not tolerate a low pH.

Sauerkraut

Cabbage (*Brassica oleraceae*), when fermented by bacteria under anaerobic conditions in the presence of salt, gives a product which has become acidified with lactic acid, known as **sauerkraut**. It is eaten by people particularly in central Europe and parts of the former USSR. Mature cabbage heads are used, with a sugar content in the range of about 2.9 to 6.4 per cent. The cabbage is washed in clean water and shredded, including even the central stalk. The shreds are mixed with about 2.5 per cent by weight of salt (sodium chloride), then packed into a vat, weighted down and covered closely. Plastic bags filled with water can be used on top, acting as a weight and a seal, but still allowing gases produced during the fermentation to escape. The salt helps to draw out moisture from the cabbage, so that the shreds become immersed in brine.

The natural flora of the cabbage includes bacterial populations which carry out the fermentation, so no starter culture is added. Respiration of the plant cells and of the bacteria soon removes the oxygen from the liquid in the container so that conditions become anaerobic. A number of different bacteria grow but gradually the acid fermenters become dominant. The salt helps because it favours the **lactic acid** bacteria. In the early stages *Enterobacter cloaca* produces some lactic acid, but the bacteria mainly responsible for the fermentation are *Leuconostoc mesenteroides* and later *Lactobacillus plantarum. Leuconostoc* ferments the sugars in the cabbage (mostly glucose and fructose) to lactic acid, to a concentration of up to 1 per cent. Carbon dioxide is given off, which helps to keep the conditions anaerobic. *Lactobacillus* is then able to utilise some of the by-products produced by *Leuconostoc*. With *Lactobacillus*, the acidity can increase to 2.0 per cent, though the best level is about 1.7 per cent lactic acid in the finished sauerkraut. This gives a pH of about 3.5. Other bacteria involved in the fermentation contribute to the flavour or lactic acid production. The temperature should be maintained above 15 °C, ideally between about 21 and 24 °C. At low temperatures, the fermentation is slow and incomplete, but if too high, undesirable fermentations by other microbes may take place.

Sausages and salami, cider, coffee and cocoa, olives, pickled herrings and mango pickle, are all examples of fermentations.
- Where were these foods originally grown and when do you think they were harvested?
- How does the fermented product differ from the original raw food – in texture and in taste? Try to find out about the microorganisms involved and the fermentation process.

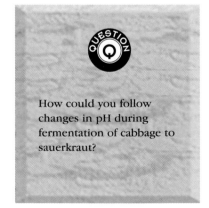

How could you follow changes in pH during fermentation of cabbage to sauerkraut?

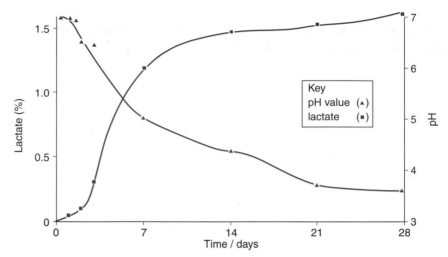

Figure 4.2 Changes in lactic acid concentration and pH during the fermentation of cabbage to sauerkraut

Vinegar

Vinegar is used world-wide, for pickling or preserving foods, as a dressing on salads, in cooking or to acidify foods and contribute to flavouring. The word *vinegar* is derived from the French *vinaigre*, meaning 'sour wine' and this hints at the means by which it is made. Vinegar is an aqueous solution (minimum 4 percent) of ethanoic acid (acetic acid). It is produced by the oxidation of ethanol. Traces of other compounds such as esters, alcohols and organic acids give variations in the flavour. The source of material used for the initial alcoholic fermentation reflects material locally available. Thus cider vinegar comes from fermentation of apple juice, wine vinegar from grape juice, malt vinegar from barley or other cereal that has undergone the malting process and rice vinegar from rice.

The first stage of the fermentation is the **anaerobic** conversion of sugar (glucose) to ethanol, and is carried out by *Saccharomyces* species (yeasts). A number of species of bacteria, known as **acetic acid bacteria**, are then involved in the **aerobic** conversion of ethanol to ethanoic acid, with ethanal (acetaldehyde) as an intermediate. These are mainly from the genera *Acetobacter* and *Gluconobacter*. Commercially, a culture of mixed strains is used. These bacteria are not killed by the low pH which develops during the process, but they are sensitive to lack of oxygen.

Traditional methods developed for the commercial production of vinegar encourage the aerobic activity of these bacteria. The simplest is the French (**Orleans**) system. A cask is filled about two-thirds full of wine and left open to the air. A film of acetic acid bacteria collects on the surface, supported by a floating wooden grid. As it forms, the vinegar is drawn off from the bottom of the cask without disturbing the film of bacteria. More wine is then added, making the process more or less continuous. This method is relatively slow, taking several weeks or months at a temperature of about 21 to 29 °C. Larger scale and quicker commercial methods are designed to increase aeration, either by **trickling** the liquid over a surface (such as wood shavings or twigs) inside a fermentation chamber, or by forced aeration within the liquid (**submerged** process). A suitable system for the trickling method is illustrated in Figure 4.3. In submerged methods, the bacteria are held in fine bubbles of air suspended in the liquid which is stirred mechanically inside a large fermentation chamber, known as an acetator.

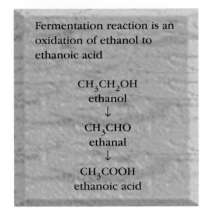

Fermentation reaction is an oxidation of ethanol to ethanoic acid

$$CH_3CH_2OH$$
ethanol
↓
$$CH_3CHO$$
ethanal
↓
$$CH_3COOH$$
ethanoic acid

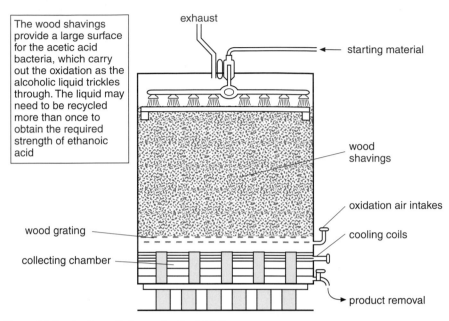

The wood shavings provide a large surface for the acetic acid bacteria, which carry out the oxidation as the alcoholic liquid trickles through. The liquid may need to be recycled more than once to obtain the required strength of ethanoic acid

exhaust

starting material

wood shavings

oxidation air intakes

cooling coils

wood grating

collecting chamber

product removal

Figure 4.3 Production of vinegar by the trickling process

The slow methods produce a high quality vinegar, whereas that produced by the quicker methods tends to have a poorer flavour. The quality can be improved by allowing the vinegar to undergo a maturation process, standing in barrels. The vinegar is generally pasteurised (see Chapter 3) by heating for a few seconds at 60 to 66 °C.

Fermented milk – yoghurt and cheese

Fermentation of milk, into yoghurt and into cheese, is both a very ancient and a widespread practice. In Europe we are most familiar with yoghurt from cow's milk, or from sheep, but milk from other mammals, including goats, buffalo and camels is also used. Probably the first yoghurt was from the Middle East. Milk being carried under warm conditions probably became sour, developed agreeable flavours and could be kept longer than fresh milk with obvious advantages to nomadic people. A portion of a successful ferment might have been used again to start the next batch, effectively selecting suitable strains of bacteria.

Yoghurt

In the modern, industrial preparation of yoghurt, whole milk may be **blended** with skimmed milk or skimmed milk solids, or starch or sugar may be added to give a different flavour or consistency. Sometimes the milk is heated to allow evaporation and make a thicker yoghurt, though on a large scale the viscosity (thickness) of the end-product is controlled by the initial mixture of milk and solids. The fat content can be adjusted by removing fat or by adding cream. The milk is **homogenised** to disperse the fat as small globules, then heated to 88 to 95 °C for between 15 and 30 minutes to **pasteurise** the milk. The high temperature and time used are necessary to kill bacteria which may be active at relatively high temperatures (described as *thermophilic* bacteria). Milk inevitably carries a microflora from the udder, and these contaminants could act as competitors in the yoghurt making process.

The starter culture includes two species of bacteria which enhance each other's activities. First, *Lactobacillus bulgaricus* acts on milk protein, converting it to small peptides and amino acids. These stimulate the growth of the second species, *Streptococcus thermophilus*. *S. thermophilus* in turn produces formic acid which stimulates growth of *L. bulgaricus*. *L. bulgaricus* is mainly responsible for the conversion of lactose to lactic acid and production of some ethanal (acetaldehyde) which, with other compounds, contributes to the flavour. The culture is incubated at 40 to 45 °C for 3 to 6 hours (or at 32 °C for 12 hours), then cooled rapidly to prevent further bacterial fermentation. At the end of the fermentation, the lactic acid concentration is about 1.4 per cent and the pH is between 4.4 and 4.6. The thickening of the yoghurt is the result of coagulation of proteins.

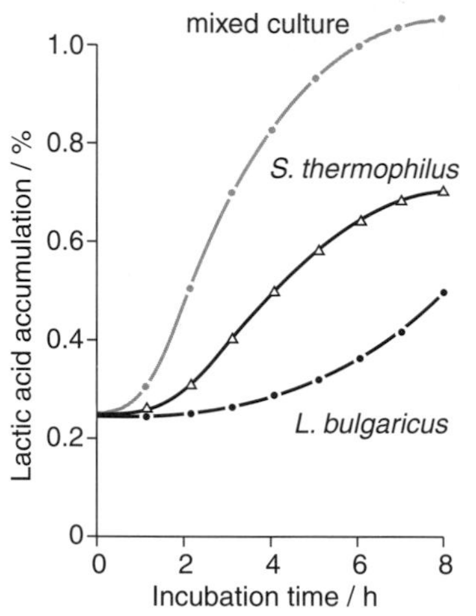

In the **set method** for making yoghurt, the homogenised milk with starter culture is poured into the final containers and incubated. More commonly, the mixture is **stirred** during the fermentation then poured into containers at the end of the process. Fruit or other flavours may be added, either at the start of incubation for set yoghurt, or at the end for stirred yoghurt. The fruit may introduce unwanted yeasts or other microbial contaminants into the yoghurt. Fruit yoghurts are often protected by adding sugar giving a higher osmotic potential and lower pH. At the same time the sugar sweetens the yoghurt. The popularity of yoghurt comes in part from its improved digestibility. Yoghurt is particularly valuable for lactose-intolerant people, but if additional milk solids are added to thicken the yoghurt, some lactose may remain in the final product. Variations in the end-product come from using cultures of different organisms.

Figure 4.4 Preparation of yoghurt and the effect of different culture organisms. Comparison of two single strain cultures, Streptococcus thermophilus *and* Lactobacillus bulgaricus, *and a mixed culture of both strains*

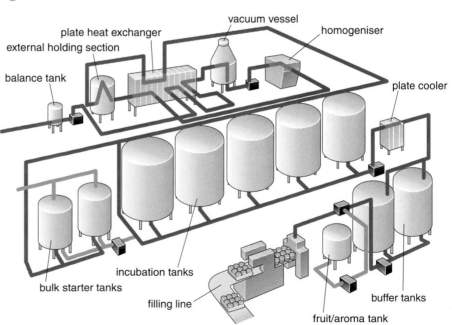

Figure 4.5 Preparation of yoghurt on an industrial scale

Cheese

Making cheese is probably the oldest way of preserving the nutrients in milk over a long period. It probably started by carrying milk in sacks made from the stomach of a sheep, cow or other domesticated mammals the people herded. Over the centuries a wide variety of traditional cheeses have developed. Differences in flavour and texture depend on the source of milk and local methods used in the later stages of treating and maturing the cheese.

The basic steps in making cheese can be summarised as follows:
- coagulation of protein in the milk to form curds
- removal of whey (a watery liquid)
- ripening or maturation (may include pressing).

It is the final step that introduces the widest range of variations in texture (soft or hard) and flavour (mild, mature, blue, etc.) to the cheese. Control of the microorganisms present is the key to the wide range of individual cheeses that are produced.

In present-day commercial production of cheese, such as English 'Cheddar' cheese, the early stages are similar to that in yoghurt-making, namely **standardisation of fat content** and **homogenisation**. The milk is then **pasteurised** by heating to 72 °C for 15 seconds, then cooled rapidly to 31 °C and transferred to the cheese vat. In the next stage, known as **ripening** (of the milk), the starter culture of lactic acid bacteria is added. This usually contains *Streptococcus lactis*, often with *S. cremoris* or other species depending on the flavour required. Conversion of lactose to lactic acid by the bacteria lowers the pH, and milk proteins (mainly casein) begin to **coagulate**. Further curd formation results from the addition of **rennet**. Traditionally this is an extract from the stomach of young calves (or from other young mammals). The active enzymes are **chymosin** (about 90 per cent) and **pepsin** (about 10 per cent). Of interest to vegetarians is the increasing use of genetically modified microorganisms to produce chymosin (see pages 72–3).

It takes about 45 minutes for the milk to clot. The curds are then separated from the liquid whey and further processed in several steps to form the cheese:
- curds cut into small pieces (about the size of a pea) – releases some whey curd heated to about 39 °C and stirred continuously to release more whey in a process known as **scalding**
- stirring is stopped, the curds settle (known as **pitching**), whey is drained off
- curd particles begin to knit together; curd is cut into large blocks which are stacked and turned – more whey drains off
- **cheddaring** involves turning and piling the blocks to achieve the desired texture. It can be done by hand or mechanically
- cutting with an electric mill (**milling**) further reduces particle size
- salt added in varying amounts – this helps to preserve the cheese and bring out desired flavours.

If making a hard cheese, the salted curd is packed into a mould and then pressed, which further reduces the water content.

A multiplicity of names are used for yoghurt-type preparations throughout the world. Find out where the following fermentations are eaten or drunk, what milk each uses, and how they differ in their processing from the yoghurt described in this chapter.
acidophilous milk; amaas; buttermilk; chal; dadih; filmjolk; kefir; kumiss; lassi; mast; raita; yakult; yiaourti

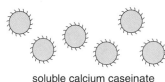

soluble calcium caseinate particles in milk

chymosin removes glycopeptides from the surface

the denuded casein particles are negatively charged and unstable

Ca²⁺ ions help particles to aggregate

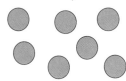

aggregated calcium paracaseinate particles in milk coagulum

Figure 4.6 Converting casein to curds – how milk protein coagulates

BIOTECHNOLOGY AND FOOD PRODUCTION

During a period of maturation, which may last up to a year or more, various enzymatic processes continue, resulting in changes in flavour and texture. Lipases convert lipids to glycerol and fatty acids – butyric acid is one that has a characteristic flavour. Proteases degrade proteins to amino acids, and in some cheeses this results in a more liquid texture. Further enzymatic action produces a variety of amines, aldehydes and ketones which contribute to the flavour. The final pH of cheeses varies from about 4.5 in cottage cheese to 6.9 in a matured camembert.

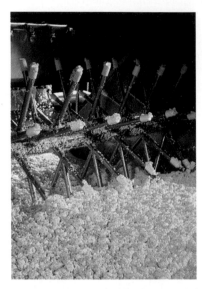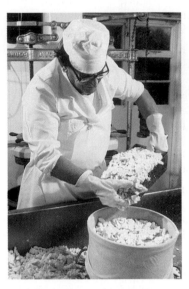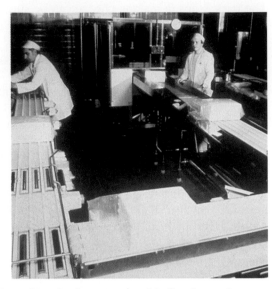

Figure 4.7 Commercial production of cheese: (a) stirring the curds on the conveyor; (b) packing the cheese into moulds (farmhouse cheese making); (c) the 'Blockformer' process - another faster method of pressing, used in mass production of cheese. The curds are taken under vacuum to the top of a vertical tower (the blockformer). As they pass down the column, further whey is removed under vacuum and pressure and the curds consolidate. At the bottom of the tower, 20kg blocks are cut off and vacuum sealed in polythene. The cross-section of the tower is the same as that of the finished block of cheese.

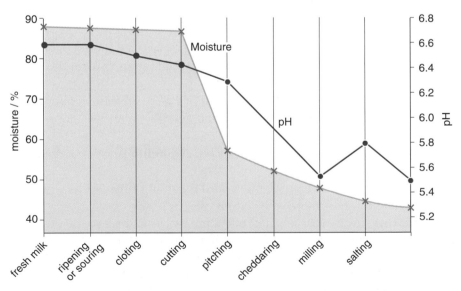

Figure 4.8 Changes in moisture and pH during the different stages of making cheddar cheese. Making cheese is essentially a dehydration process, allowing the fat and casein in the milk to be concentrated to 5 or 10 times their original. Fermentation of lactose to lactic acid contributes to the lowering of the pH

Table 4.1 *Features of some cheese varieties – differences in the type of milk, the microorganisms used in the fermentation or ripening stages, the extent of dehydration and the time for maturation have led to the development of hundreds or thousands of local cheese varieties*

Type	Examples	Features
very hard	Parmesan	made from semi-skimmed cow's milk, pressed, dried and matured for 1 to 4 years
hard	Cheddar, Leicester Cheshire Gruyere, Emmental (Swiss cheeses)	see text for description – matured 6 to 12 months more crumbly than cheddar, matured 3 to 6 months carbon dioxide produced by bacteria collects in pockets, giving the characteristic holes
semi-hard (white)	Lancashire, Wensleydale	whole cow'smilk used, matured 1 to 4 months; mild flavour; crumbly
semi-hard (white-brined)	Feta	from cow, sheep or goat milk; matured in brine for 3 to 10 weeks
semi-hard (blue)	Gorgonzola, Roquefort (sheep), Stilton (cow)	cow, sheep, or goat milk used (for Gorgonzola); thr mould Penicillium roqueforti added to curds before removing the whey; mould grows through the cheese; fungal spores give the blue colour; characteristic flavour due to enzymatic conversion of fats to fatty acids and ketones
soft	Cottage cheese Brie, Camembert Mozzarella	high moisture; unripen; eaten fresh high moisture; surface ripened due to mould and bacterial growth from buffalo or cow milk; curd pulled to long pliable mass; eaten fresh or after 1 to 2 weeks

Table 4.2 *Nutrient content of different types of cheese*

Nutrient	Type of cheese – composition as g per 100 g				
	Cheddar	Cheshire	Cheddar-like reduced fat cheese	Surface mould ripened cheese	Cottage cheese
water	37.5	42.0	46.0	42.0	78.8
total fat	34.4	31.4	15.0	40.0	4.0
(of which saturates)	22.0	20.1	9.0	23.9	92.4
protein	25.5	24.0	29.5	16.0	13.6
carbohydrate	0.08	0.11	<0.2	<0.2	1.4
calcium / mg	736	540	860	470	60
vitamin A / µg	340	344	107	358	35
riboflavin / mg	0.42	0.48	0.60	0.42	0.19
vitamin D / µg	0.26	0.26	0.12	0.31	0.02
energy / KJ 100 g–1	1705	1570	1059	1752	402

Soya bean products – soya milk, tofu, soya sauce

The soya (soy) bean, *Glycine max*, is a legume, grown widely on a global scale. It is valued as a food because of its high protein content, as well as for its oil and vitamins. Soya bean products are particularly important in Oriental diets, and have probably been utilised in China for 4000 years or more. Mature soya beans, if eaten raw, are toxic and have an unpleasant taste, but when cooked or further processed have given rise to a whole range of different foods. Different names are given to the products, depending on the country of origin and the local method of preparation.

Curds . . . and whey – waste it or use it?

Whey is a by-product of the cheese industry. It contains about 5 per cent lactose and less than 1 per cent of non-casein proteins. It could be wasted, but there is increasing interest in using it to manufacture other commercial products. One process uses the enzyme lactase, immobilised on glass beads, to produce sugars and syrups which are then used in the confectionery industry for soft-centred chocolates and for cake icings. In Eastern Europe whey is fermented to Prokllada for a sweet or a savoury drink.

- What environmental problems could arise if waste whey was discharged from factories into nearby waterways?
  Which sugars are produced from lactose and what are the advantages of using immobilised enzymes in commercial manufacturing processes?

BIOTECHNOLOGY AND FOOD PRODUCTION

Soya products are important in traditional Oriental diets. Bean curd can, for example, be fermented into a form of cheese, or dried and made into a paste. In China, cow's milk is not readily available and soya milk has been used as a substitute for human milk for feeding infants.

Suggest why cow's milk is not part of the diet in much of China.

Can you think of some reasons why soya milk is now being sold increasingly in European supermarkets?

Soya milk and **tofu** are the simplest foods derived from soya beans. The milk is obtained by mixing the soya beans with water and grinding them to a slurry which is then boiled and filtered. The filtrate is known as soya milk. When calcium sulphate, magnesium sulphate or vinegar is added, the proteins coagulate to give the bean curd. The whey (liquid) is discarded. The bean curd is bland in taste, though it can be made into a range of foods with different uses in the diet.

Preparation of **soya sauce** uses soya beans together with a starchy crop, often wheat. There are several stages in the process. The soya beans are soaked in water, boiled and drained. The starch material is added as a flour or meal – wheat, for example, may be roasted then crushed before addition. The mixture is spread on trays and a starter culture is introduced. This culture contains a mixture of moulds and bacteria and is either prepared freshly or carried over from a previous fermentation. The mixture ferments for about 1 week, at a temperature of 28 to 30 °C. The activity is mainly due to the mould *Aspergillus oryzae (soyae)* which produces amylases and proteases. The action of these enzymes results in the formation of simple sugars and amino acids which are then metabolised by other microorganisms in the later stages of the fermentation. Brine as a solution of 17–22 per cent sodium chloride, is then added and the mash is transferred to large vats. Bacteria involved in this second stage of fermentation include *Bacillus, Lactobacillus* and *Pediococcus* species. These contribute to a lowering of the pH, partly due to lactic acid production. The yeast *Saccharomyces rouxii* is responsible for production of some alcohol and development of flavour compounds. This fermentation occurs at a temperature of between 25 and 33 °C and continues for a few months or even up to a year. When mature, the dark brown liquid soya sauce is filtered off and usually pasteurised. Variations in flavour can be achieved by altering the fermentation conditions or microorganisms present in the culture.

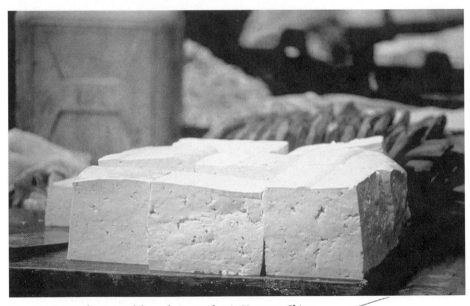

Figure 4.9 Soya bean curd for sale in market in Yunnan, China

Bread – from wheat flour

Today most bread is made from wheat flour, though rye and other flours can be used. A simple, unleavened (flat) bread can be made by mixing flour with water then baking it. Using yeast in the mixture produces the lighter, leavened bread, now consumed widely throughout the world. The yeast used by bakers is a suitably selected strain of *Saccharomyces cerevisiae*. The process requires mixing of flour with water, salt and yeast and often some sugar is added. Enzymes (α and β amylases) in the wheat flour hydrolyse amylose and amylopectin in the starch, mainly to maltose and some glucose. The yeast utilises the sugars, converting them to carbon dioxide and some ethanol. The carbon dioxide is responsible for the raising of the bread dough. As the gas expands it becomes trapped in the dough, making it lighter.

During the mixing, or **kneading**, the dough kept at a temperature of about 26 °C. At first the yeast grows and produces carbon dioxide. In a second kneading, the dough is 'knocked back', letting some gas escape and causing the dough to tighten up. It is then cut and put into tins or moulds for baking. Typically the whole process of 'proving' the dough can take up to 4 hours. On **baking** at about 232 °C for 15 minutes or longer (depending on the type of loaf), the carbon dioxide is expelled, leaving holes in the hardened dough, and the ethanol escapes. The high temperatures kill the yeast preventing further action.

The secret to the structure of the bread lies in the properties of the proteins in wheat flour. Collectively the proteins are called glutens, made up mostly of gliadin and glutenin. A good bread flour, described as 'hard', has a protein content of 10 to 14 per cent, whereas softer flour has a protein content below 10 per cent and is more suitable for making biscuits or pastry. When the water is mixed with the flour, the proteins absorb water to form an elastic gluten complex. This allows the dough to stretch and retain the bubbles of carbon dioxide. The strength of the gluten is derived from the way the long, branched protein chains link together, to form a sort of network. This is enhanced by links between –SH (sulphydryl) groups from the amino acid cysteine, forming long, branched chains which give the dough its strength. The kneading process is important for several reasons – it mixes the ingredients allowing even dispersion of the carbon dioxide bubbles, but also plays a part in the modification of the proteins, allowing the chains to line up alongside each other and form the cross-links.

Improvers such as **ascorbic acid** (vitamin C), are sometimes added to bread flour to speed up the processing time. During the intense mixing, the ascorbic acid is oxidised to dehydroascorbic acid. It then interacts with the –SH groups by removing hydrogen and forming disulphide S–S bridges very rapidly. This helps the dough structure to form and tighten quickly, giving a reduced fermentation time. Large-scale commercial bread-making processes also utilise higher levels of yeast. Other improvers have been used to bleach flour to make it whiter, though consumer preferences are now swinging in favour of unbleached flour.

Tempe is an Indonesian fermented food, made from soya beans. It is now being produced more widely in other parts of the world. Why do you think tempe is an important part of the diet for Indonesians? Find out which mould is responsible for the fermentation and how you could carry out this fermentation. [You will find help in the National Centre for Biotechnology Education (NCBE) practical guides.]

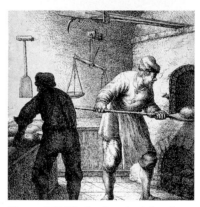

Figure 4.10 The basic principle of breadmaking have changed little. This engraving shows a baker making bread in 1635.

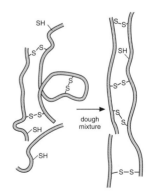

Figure 4.11 Bread dough and the kneading process. Molecular changes in the gluten proteins and the formation of cross-links between sulphydryl groups contribute to the properties of the dough which enable it to trap carbon dioxide gas

Wine making

Making wine ranks as one of the oldest, and perhaps most pleasurable, of biotechnologies, enjoyed by countless individuals and with an important influence on successive cultures over the centuries. It is not difficult to see how a pile of surplus, discarded fruit began to ferment, and the liquor which seeped out was enjoyed for its flavour and alcoholic effects. Three thousand years ago the Greeks savoured wine which was kept in large pottery vessels. They later used barrels lined with pine resin – this increased storage time and allowed the wine to mature. The art of making wine has spread from the vineyards of Europe to world-wide production and consumption. Today, wine is generally understood to mean the alcoholic fermentation by yeast of sugars in grapes, from the vine *Vitis vinifera*, though wines are made from other fruits, vegetables or grains, such as apple, date, elderberry, parsnip and rice, as well as flowers, which contribute to the 'bouquet' of the wine. The fermentation of wine from grapes is described here, though similar principles apply to the production of other alcoholic beverages.

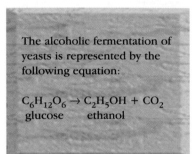

The alcoholic fermentation of yeasts is represented by the following equation:

$$C_6H_{12}O_6 \rightarrow C_2H_5OH + CO_2$$
$$\text{glucose} \qquad \text{ethanol}$$

Wild yeasts naturally present on the skins of grapes can contribute to the fermentation, but in commercial production selected strains of a wine yeast are used, usually *Saccharomyces cerevisiae var ellipsoideus*. Such yeasts show some tolerance to the level of alcohol produced, though this inhibits the growth of many other microorganisms. Initially respiration is aerobic, but as oxygen is depleted, the yeast switches to anaerobic respiration. There is then less growth of the yeast but the sugars are fermented to ethanol. Towards the end of the fermentation, lactic acid bacteria may ferment malic acid to lactic acid. Other bacteria may also contribute to the development of flavours in the later stages, during ageing or maturation.

The main stages in the production of wine can be summarised as follows:
- crushing of the fruit to make a **must**, followed by separation of the juice
- fermentation with yeast
- racking to draw off the clear wine
- ageing and maturation.

Grapes are harvested when they have the desired sugar content, generally between 15 and 25 percent. The sugars are mainly glucose and fructose. Another important component is the acid content, consisting mainly of malic and tartaric acids. The sugar–acid balance is influenced by the variety of grape and the conditions under which it has grown. The grapes are removed from their stems, crushed mechanically and the juice pressed out. Treatment with sulphur dioxide prevents further growth of wild yeasts, or of bacteria which may lead to souring of the wine by converting it to vinegar. Sometimes the juice is pasteurised by heating to 85 °C for a short time instead of using the sulphite treatment. Yeast is added to the juice in large tanks or fermenting vats. For white wine, the skins and pips are removed, but for red wine a proportion of the skins of black grapes are retained. Pigments in the skins contribute to the red colour and tannins give a characteristic taste.

For the first few days, the contents of the tank are mixed by pushing the 'cap' of floating skins and other debris into the tank of juice. This keeps the conditions aerobic and encourages growth of the yeast. The mixing is then stopped to allow anaerobic conditions to develop so that fermentation to ethanol occurs. For white wines, the temperature is maintained at about 10 to 20 °C and the fermentation takes about 7 to 14 days. For red wine, the fermentation is carried out at temperatures between 24 and 27 °C for about 3 to 5 days. Heat is released during the fermentation so there must be a means of cooling to prevent adverse conditions. At higher temperatures, some of the lactobacilli and other microorganisms grow successfully and compete with the yeast. At lower temperatures, a number of volatile compounds are produced which contribute to the flavour of a particular wine, but if the temperature is too low, activity of the wine yeast is reduced and other microorganisms may predominate, with undesirable results. During the fermentation, carbon dioxide accumulates above the liquid, helping to keep conditions anaerobic.

After the first stage of fermentation, the wine is **racked**, or drawn off from the residue, known as lees. Racking may be repeated several times before the fermentation is completed. In a dry wine, all the sugar will be utilised and converted to alcohol, whereas in sweeter wines, some sugar remains. A high initial sugar content is likely to lead to a higher alcohol content, though there comes a point at which yeasts can no longer tolerate increases in alcohol content. Some wines are artificially sweetened by addition of sugar at an early stage. For sparkling wines, including champagne, further sucrose and yeast can be added to initiate a secondary fermentation in the bottles. Bubbles of carbon dioxide held in the wine give the sparkling or gassy effect. In some cases, carbon dioxide is added artificially.

The fermented wine is often cloudy, though it becomes clearer on standing and after racking. At a late stage, a process known as **fining** may be carried out, which involves the addition of materials which adsorb the suspended particles and help them to settle. Some wines are pasteurised at this stage or sulphur dioxide may be added. Finally the wine is allowed to age, either in the bottle or preferably in oak barrels. Further chemical reactions take place, resulting in the development of different flavours. The wood or cork allows some access of oxygen leading to oxidation reactions which contribute to these flavours. Fortified wines (such as port, sherry and vermouth) are made by adding spirit (often brandy). This increases the alcoholic content and prevents further activity of yeasts or other microorganisms.

A recipe for home-made apple wine requires 10 kg of apples, 1.5 kg of sugar per 4.5 litres of liquor, 4.5 litres of water, yeast and nutrient. The recipe reads as follows: "Chop the apples into small pieces, put into a bucket, add the yeast, nutrient and water. Leave for about a week, stirring vigorously several times a day to bring the apples at the bottom to the top. Keep the bucket closely covered and in a fairly warm place. Then strain the juice from the apple pulp. Press the juice from the apples and add to the rest of the liquor. To every 4.5 litres add 1.5 kg of sugar. Put into cask or glass fermenting vessel and fit air-lock, racking when it has cleared. The wine will be ready for drinking within six months, but improves with keeping for up to a year." Why are the apples chopped into small pieces? Why is the wine stirred vigorously for the first few days? Typically the nutrient contains ammonium, phosphate and sulphate. Why do you think it is added? Why is the bucket kept covered and in a warm place? What do you expect to be happening while the chopped apples are in the bucket? Why is it possible to press the juice out after a week but not at the beginning? Why is the sugar added, and what happens if less, or more sugar is added? What is meant by *racking*? Why does the wine improve on keeping? Why are wine-makers advised to keep utensils as clean and sterile as possible? Find out the difference between making wine and cider. Why do you think cider is a golden brown colour? Incidentally, using this recipe, 25 kg of apples make about 25 litres of wine. After pressing, the apple pulp left forms into a cake measuring only 10 cm deep and 25 cm in diameter!

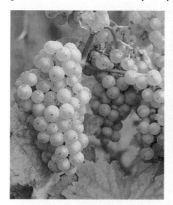
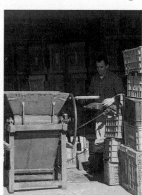
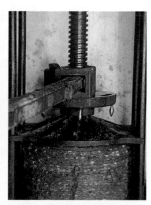

Figure 4.12 Wine making: (a) grapes growing in a Suffolk vineyard (England); (b) harvested grapes being crushed in Andalucia (Spain); (c) a simple press used to release the juice from the crushed grapes in Andalucia (Spain).

BIOTECHNOLOGY AND FOOD PRODUCTION

Devise a series of flow charts which summarise the stages in the processes of the fermentations described in this chapter – for making sauerkraut, vinegar, yoghurt and cheese, soya sauce, making dough from flour and then baking it to form bread, and making wine. Remember to include the microorganisms as well as the necessary conditions.

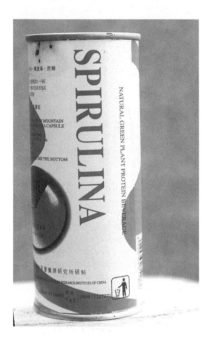

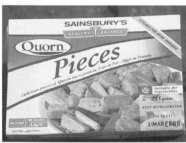

Figure 4.13 (a) A 'natural green plant protein beverage' - drink containing Spirulina *produced and for sale in SW China; (b) mycoprotein - marketed as Quorn® - on sale in the UK*

Microorganisms as food

Single-cell protein (SCP) and mycoprotein

The term single-cell protein (SCP) is used to describe protein derived from microbial cells (such as yeasts, other fungi, algae and bacteria), though the microorganism producing the protein is not necessarily 'single-celled'. The whole organism is harvested and consumed, rather than using the products of their fermentations or other processing. Exploitation of SCP production offers a way of increasing the available protein for consumption by livestock and by humans, and could be valuable, particularly in areas where the land is infertile or the climate inhospitable. While SCP production may have potential for feeding the ever-increasing world population, in practice only a few schemes have proved to be commercially successful. Photosynthetic organisms include *Spirulina maxima*, which is grown in open ponds or basins.

Table 4.3 lists some of the perceived advantages of SCP production, and some of the disadvantages that have come to light with industrial schemes already attempted. The most successful microbial food for human consumption has been mycoprotein, marketed under the name of Quorn®. It is obtained from growth of the fungus *Fusarium graminearum*, using food-grade glucose syrup as the carbon source, gaseous ammonia for nitrogen and added salts. Other SCP products are given in Table 4.4. In developing commercial schemes, palatability is an important feature if it is to be used for human consumption, or ways must be found to incorporate the SCP into familiar foods to increase protein content. Ultimately the success depends on the economics of microbial production compared with protein production from animals and plants in conventional agriculture and horticulture.

Table 4.3 Single-cell protein – some advantages and disadvantages

Advantages of SCP
• fast growth rate, high yield in relatively short time
• production throughout the year, regardless of season
• range of substrates can be utilised, including waste materials from industrial processes
• high protein content compared with some other sources (such as soya bean or fish meal)

Disadvantages of SCP
• may be deficient in certain amino acids, such as methionine or other sulphur-containing amino acids, which are essential for humans or other animals
• microbial cell walls indigestible by humans and non-ruminant animals
• the high RNA content in mocrobial cells unsuitable for humans because they lack the enzyme which would break it down
• concern that toxins may persist in the growth medium when using wastes from industrial purposes

Use of DNA (gene) technology in food production

Chymosin

In cheese-making, **chymosin** (rennin) is the main enzyme involved in the coagulation of casein, the protein in milk. Traditionally, the source of chymosin was usually **rennet**, an extract from the fourth stomach (the abomasum) of

Table 4.4 Microorganisms as food – some attempts to utilise SCP

Microorganism	Substrate used	Product, use, comments
Fusarium graminearum (filamentous fungus)	glucose syrup + gaseous ammonia, salts, biotin	mycoprotein, filamentous fungus, texture similar to meat products
Candida lipolytica (yeast)	alkanes (n-paraffin) + supply of gaseous ammonia, phosphate, other salts	alkanes Toprina-G, used as feed additive – no longer made
Methylophilus methylotrophus (bacterium)	methanol + ammonia, phosphate, other salts	'Pruteen' for animal feed – no longer made
Spirulina sp. (blue -green bacterium)	photosynthesis – grown in open ponds	dried and fed to animals, becoming popular as a 'health food', eaten by people around Lake Chad in Africa, also by Aztecs in ancient Mexico

young calves, or sometimes from kids or lambs. In the 16th century, rennet was prepared by cutting strips of the stomach of young calves and steeping these in warm milk or brine to extract the rennet. By the late 19th century the first industrial preparation of calf rennet was established by a Danish chemist. Calves destined for consumption as veal were used, so they were not sacrificed specifically for extraction of the enzyme. More recently, in the 1960s, because of changing eating patterns, there was concern that there would be a world-wide shortage of rennet for commercial cheese production. This led to pressure to find alternative sources of rennet and to develop substitutes to keep up with the demand.

Bovine rennet from adult cattle can be used as an alternative to calf chymosin, but the bovine extract contains a higher proportion of pepsin and gives a lower yield of cheese. Certain fungi produce proteases which can clot milk proteins. **Fungal enzymes** are now used in more than one third of cheese produced world-wide. Three fungi used for production of the enzymes are *Mucor miehei*, *M. pusillus* and *Endothia parasitica*. Compared with calf chymosin, the fungal enzymes are more stable, but this can be a disadvantage in cheeses which have a long maturing stage (e.g. Cheddar cheese) because degradation of the milk proteins continues. To counteract this, these enzymes can be destabilised, using oxidising agents, so that they behave in a way similar to the more successful calf chymosin. Fungal enzymes are used widely in production of vegetarian cheese.

DNA technology has provided further substitutes for calf rennet. The first microorganisms capable of making chymosin were produced in 1981, using *Escherichia coli*. Now chymosin is produced from genetically modified yeasts, including *Kluyveromyces lactis* and *Saccharomyces cerevisiae*. Precisely the same DNA code as in the calf is incorporated into the microorganism, so the enzyme produced is identical to that from calves. Expert tasters can detect no differences between the cheeses produced using chymosin from genetically modified organisms and that from extracted calf rennet. The enzymes actually

A quick brew of questions about fermentations – a chance to look back over each one described.
Aerobic or anaerobic
Which fermentations occur under aerobic conditions and which under anaerobic?
How is the aeration (or lack of it) maintained during the fermentation?
Lactic acid for preservation
Which fermentations produce lactic acid?
How low does the pH become in these various fermentations?
Texture and taste
Which proteins are altered during the fermentation, giving a change in texture, in yoghurt, in cheese and in bread?
What about soya products?
Why is yoghurt runny but cheese solid and sometimes hard?
List some of the organic compounds which contribute to flavours in the end product, in any of these fermentations.
Additives
Why is salt added to cabbage when making sauerkraut?
Why are sugar and ascorbic acid added to flour in bread-making?
Why is sulphite (or sulphur dioxide) added at an early stage of wine making and why is it sometimes added to the wine before bottling?
Bug or bugs
Under natural conditions – such as alcoholic fermentation of fruit juices – a number of microorganisms may contribute to the fermentation, but in commercial production, a starter culture of one, two or more selected strains of microbe is often used. Which fermentations use wild populations of microbes?
Which cultures have only one species of microbe, and which have two, three or more?
How do these different microorganisms interact with each other?
How is interspecific competition from unwanted microbes avoided during the fermentation?
Why do we use a starter culture of selected strains?

have fewer impurities and their behaviour is more predictable. At first there was resistance to accepting cheese made with the involvement of genetically modified organisms (GMOs). Before being released for general consumption, there was rigorous testing of the products. The enzymes used for cheese produced in this way have been approved by the relevant regulatory bodies and by the Vegetarian Society. Such cheese is on sale in a number of countries, including the UK.

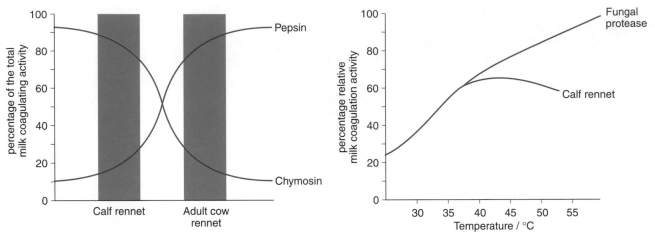

Figure 4.14 (a)Changes in relative proportions of chymosin and pepsin with age of calf to adult; (b) Differences in behaviour of calf rennet and fungal protease – influence of temperature

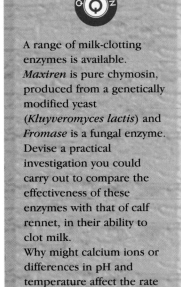

QUESTION

A range of milk-clotting enzymes is available. *Maxiren* is pure chymosin, produced from a genetically modified yeast (*Kluyveromyces lactis*) and *Fromase* is a fungal enzyme. Devise a practical investigation you could carry out to compare the effectiveness of these enzymes with that of calf rennet, in their ability to clot milk.

Why might calcium ions or differences in pH and temperature affect the rate of setting of the curds?

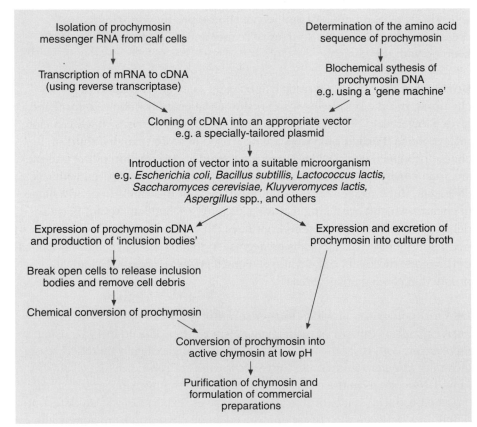

Figure 4.15 Stages in the production of calf chymosin by genetically modified microorganisms. Prochymosin is an inactive precursor of chymosin

Genetically modified tomatoes

There is something both irresistible and alluring about a freshly picked, ripe, home-grown tomato. The characteristic smell, texture and rich, sweet flavour, whether eaten raw or cooked to a simple sauce, are rarely experienced in mass-produced supermarket tomatoes. This is hardly surprising. Commercial tomato growers are geared to large-scale production. The priorities are to maximise yield and to minimise losses through disease. Production and harvest time are geared to consumer demand. The tomatoes are expected to be uniform in size and to arrive undamaged on the supermarket shelf. Flavour is not always high on the list of priorities. Often tomatoes are picked when they are green and unripe which means they are firm enough to survive the handling during harvesting, storage and distribution. To some extent the ripening stages can be controlled, so that pre-packed boxes of red tomatoes reach the displays on the supermarket shelves.

Tomatoes soften as they ripen, mainly because of the activity of the enzyme polygalacturonase (PG) (see Chapter 3). PG acts on pectic substances in the middle lamella within the cell wall structure, hydrolysing long polymers and converting them to shorter more soluble fragments. The cells lose their cohesion, so begin to move in relation to each other. Turgor of the cells diminishes as the cell walls weaken, resulting in loss of firmness. Synthesis of PG coincides with the rise in ethene concentration. Inhibition of PG activity slows the softening but still allows development of the desirable flavours and colour associated with ripening..

Genetic modification, using two different methods, has led to a precise way of reducing the expression of the PG gene so that the tomato remains firm. The gene that codes for PG has been identified and sequenced. Using *Agrobacterium* as a vector, an 'antisense' PG gene has been inserted into the tomato plant (see Figure 4.17). An antisense gene is effectively a reversed form of the gene and is inherited in a normal Mendelian way. Transgenic tomatoes produced by antisense technology have been approved for sale in the USA, under the name of '*Flavr-Savr*'. Research in the UK has produced genetically modified tomatoes with a shortened PG gene (Figure 4.17). In the UK, approval for the sale of paste (but not the fresh fruit) made from these genetically modified tomatoes was given in 1995. As well as improved flavour, these tomatoes show improvements in consistency and viscosity, giving a thicker tomato paste, without the need for addition of thickeners. There is much less wastage in the field at harvest and in the processing.

Genetically modified crop plants and products – social and ethical implications

In this chapter we have described the processes involved in fermentation of traditional foods, such as yoghurt and cheese, bread, wine and vinegar. It is, however, convenient to distinguish between traditional fermentations and more recent developments in biotechnology concerned with genetic modification. Development of techniques which enable the modification of DNA means that scientists can, in a very precise way, alter the genome within an organism or transfer genes, or segments of genes, from one organism to

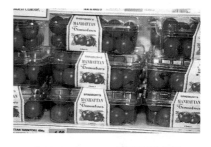

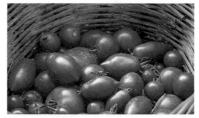

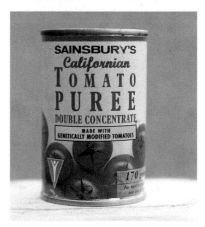

Figure 4.16 (a) Tomatoes on sale in a supermarket - selected for their size and uniformity, stored to ensure controlled ripeness on the supermarket shelf; (b) a basketful of home-grown tomatoes - rich red in colour, variable in size and shape and picked when ripe, ready to eat and full of flavour; (c) tomato paste made from genetically modified tomatoes.

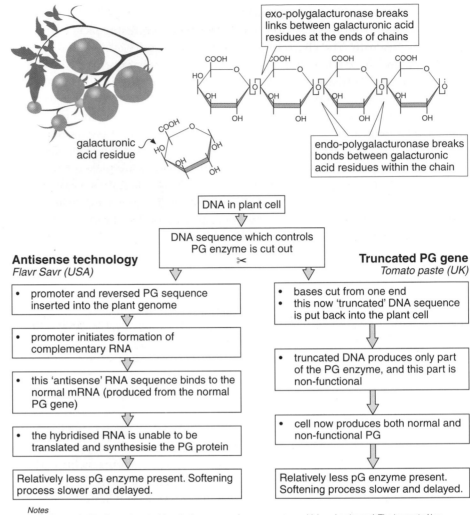

exo-polygalacturonase breaks links between galacturonic acid residues at the ends of chains

galacturonic acid residue

endo-polygalacturonase breaks bonds between galacturonic acid residues within the chain

DNA in plant cell

DNA sequence which controls PG enzyme is cut out

Antisense technology
Flavr Savr (USA)

Truncated PG gene
Tomato paste (UK)

- promoter and reversed PG sequence inserted into the plant genome

- promoter initiates formation of complementary RNA

- this 'antisense' RNA sequence binds to the normal mRNA (produced from the normal PG gene)

- the hybridised RNA is unable to be translated and synthesisie the PG protein

Relatively less pG enzyme present. Softening process slower and delayed.

- bases cut from one end
- this now 'truncated' DNA sequence is put back into the plant cell

- truncated DNA produces only part of the PG enzyme, and this part is non-functional

- cell now produces both normal and non-functional PG

Relatively less pG enzyme present. Softening process slower and delayed.

Notes

1 **Antisense technology** - A normal functioning gene produces a message which makes 'sense'. The 'promoter' is a DNA sequence at the beginning of the gene which promotes transcription of the gene, producing the mRNA from the DNA strand. Antisense technology inserts the promoter and the sequence of DNA into the genome of the plant cell, but at a different position and reserves the orientation. This DNA sequence now produces 'antisense' mRNA which is complementary to the normal sense RNA. These complementary strands of RNA bind together, so making the mRNA non-functional in terms of synthesising the relevant protein.

2 You will see that no 'foreign' DNA has been introduced into the tomatoes. In both methods, the genetic modification has been achieved by manipulation of the tomato plant's own DNA.

Figure 4.17 Two different methods of genetic modification

another. The modified organism can be engineered to produce a particular protein, or certain metabolic processes could be altered deliberately. In a transgenic organism, DNA from a different species has been incorporated into the genome. This means, for example, that a human gene could be inserted into a bacterium or yeast, or a bacterial gene could be inserted into a crop plant – in other words, the species barrier can be crossed.

The techniques of genetic modification are now also applied to breeding of plants and animals. For centuries, farmers have modified their plant crops and their domesticated animals. They have done this by the slow processes of breeding and selection of desired characteristics in the progeny and have thereby manipulated the gene pool and achieved considerable improvement in varieties used. Examples of such improvements include increased yields and refinement of texture or flavour. Animals have become more docile, the fat content of meat and in milk has been reduced, and modern wheat grown for bread yields far more viable grain than the ancestral types. Modern biotechnology carries conventional methods of breeding and artificial selection a stage further. With its 'cut and paste' techniques, DNA technology (gene technology) allows much more precise control of the specific genes that are incorporated into the genome and success is likely to be achieved in a much shorter time.

In the food industry, there is enormous potential for applications of DNA technology, bringing improvements in crop plants and products from microorganisms. Some of the aims in current research programmes are outlined in Table 4.5. The few examples below illustrate a selection of the achievements up to 1997, though in this active field of research, the pattern changes fast. The production of **chymosin for cheese making** from genetically modified yeasts and the story behind **genetically modified tomatoes** are described on page 75.

Table 4.5 *Current research with genetically modified crop plants and possible benefits*

Feature in genetically modified organism	Possible benefits
improve efficiency of uptake of mineral salts	reduced fertiliser input
improve ability to withstand drought or high salt	crop cultivated on land where soil or climate is normally unsuitable
improve resistance to herbicides	crop better able to survive application of herbicides to control weeds
improve resistance to disease	reduced pesticide input, reduced crop losses
improve frost resistance	extended growing and harvest season
control ripening of fruits	reduced postharvest losses

- **Rice and resistance to disease:** rice is a very important crop on a global scale, but suffers from the rice stripe virus (RSV). Transgenic rice, produced by introducing the gene for the virus protein coat into the rice plant genome, shows noticeably increased resistance to the rice stripe virus.
- **Maize and resistance to pests:** maize is used for human and for animal food and may be processed to provide flour, oil, syrups or other food ingredients. The European Corn Borer (ECB) is a pest which destroys around 4 per cent of maize crops on a global scale and up to 20 per cent in some regions. The pest causes damage by boring through the stem and ear of the maize plant, which then falls over. Genetically modified maize has been produced which shows resistance to pests. The pest-resistant maize produces a lethal protein when attacked by the insect. The gene for this toxic protein comes from *Bacillus thuringiensis*, which is already used widely as a biological control agent. This protein is toxic to a variety of insects but not to animals and humans.
- **Soya and herbicide resistance**: processed soya beans are used in many foods, to provide protein, oil and other ingredients. Varieties of genetically modified soya have been developed which are more tolerant to certain herbicides. The herbicides used break down relatively quickly in the soil into harmless components. The processed GM soya is shown to be indistinguishable from conventional soya in its composition and processing characteristics.

Cut and paste techniques with DNA
Different techniques are used in the manipulation of DNA. Find out what you can about the following techniques:
- gene synthesis and the polymerase chain reaction
- using plasmids as vectors
- gene ballistics
- electroporation
- microinjection of DNA (into newly fertilised eggs)
- cell fusion.

What organisms is each technique used for – plant, animal or microbe? You will get some help from *Cell Biology and Genetics*.

• **Wheat for bread-making:** strong flour for bread-making requires both elasticity and extensibility in the gluten proteins to form a good dough which will trap the carbon dioxide. Wheat grown in the UK has glutens with low elasticity, but genes have been inserted to give improved gluten proteins and a better quality bread.

The benefits of DNA technology can be viewed in a wider context. Increased resistance to disease reduces crop losses but there are additional environmental as well as economic benefits through reducing dependence on chemical pesticides. Slower or controlled ripening of fruits, or firmer but ripe tomatoes, means better quality for the consumer, as well as reduced postharvest crop losses. Improved frost resistance in strawberries could extend the growing season and hence the availability of fresh produce for the consumer. The possibilities of applying DNA technology and tapping of genetic resources could have a greater impact than the so-called Green Revolution, of the 1960s and 1970s, which relied upon the intensive input of fertilisers, pesticides and herbicides. In the face of escalating world population, biotechnology gives considerable hope to people in developing countries to overcome the shortfall in food production.

Figure 4.18 Improvement in wheat plants (a) Conventional plant breeding has produced varieties of wheat with different stem length – the shorter, stronger stems help prevent the wheat plants from being blown over in wet, windy conditions; (b) Improved bread flour from genetically modified wheat plants. Genes for high molecular weight polypeptides (HMW) have been transferred experimentally into certain wheat cultivars and the bread made from this flour (left) has a lighter, spongier texture than that produced from flour low in HMW

The impact of modern biotechnology raises issues beyond just the science and technology. A common initial reaction to DNA technology is that it is 'unnatural', 'interfering with nature'. There is the feeling that people have gained too much control over the fate and future of living organisms, that they are 'playing God'. For some religious groups there is belief in the fixity of created species, and such people find it difficult to accept any sort of interference or manipulation at the genetic level. There are suggestions that biotechnology involves taking risks for commercial gain, and that the biotechnology companies benefit rather than some of the economically vulnerable communities in the world. These are ethical and moral concerns and arouse strong and different emotions in people. The debate is carried out by a chain of people involved in the decision making – those responsible for the original research, the field trials, the food companies and retailers with their marketing strategies through to the consumer or wider public, and the regulators who scrutinise the development at every stage.

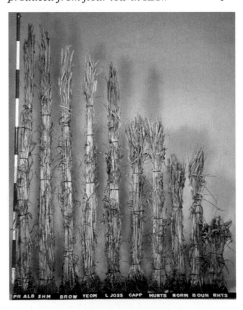

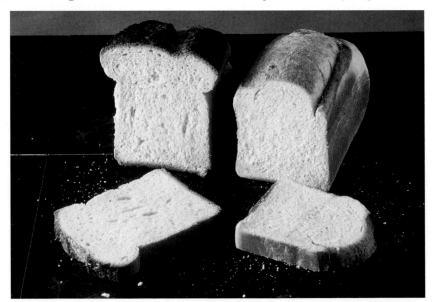

There are fears that release of GMOs could be directly harmful to humans (or other organisms), or disturb the ecological balance and natural interaction between organisms – a balance that has evolved over a long period of time. Less extreme is the possibility of 'biological pollution' – that GMOs, once released, will spread and compete with or destroy existing wild populations.

For lay people, not directly involved with science or with the food technology industry, there are varying degrees of awareness of biotechnology, and of DNA technology in particular. Reservations about DNA technology are stronger when it has been applied to food or to farm animals, but acceptance is greater in the field of medicine or involving plants (Table 4.6). For some people, the concerns about DNA technology stem from their unfamiliarity with the processes, and uncertainty about the effective control of the technology. In one supermarket chain in the UK, over three quarters of a million cans of GM tomato paste were sold between its introduction in February 1996, up to November 1997. The cans were clearly labelled to indicate the paste had been made with GM tomatoes and the conventional equivalent was always available alongside. In some stores, sales of the GM paste exceeded that of the conventional paste.

Table 4.6 *Public attitudes to gene technology – some opinions*
(a) Data from a study in Europe in 1987. "On a scale 1 to 10 where 1 is totally unacceptable and 10 is totally acceptable, where would you rank 'genetic manipulation of . . . .?'" Responses give average acceptability of genetic manipulation of cells from:

Human	Other	Bacteria	Plant
4.5	5.3	5.6	6.6

(b) Support for applications of biotechnology Eurobarometer 1991 & 1993 (from +2 = definitely agree to –2 = definitely disagree)

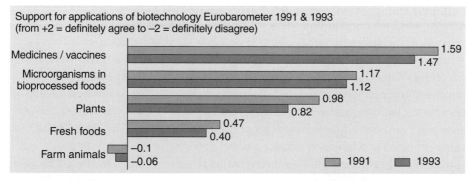

(c) Data from a study in Europe in 1991. The question asked was: "Science and technology change the way we live. Do you think that biotechnology and genetic engineering will improve our way of life in the next 20 years, it will have no effect, or will it make things worse?"

Response	B	DK	D	GR	SP	F	IR	I	L	N	UK
Will improve	49.2	43.6	43.7	39.1	57.9	53.7	48.4	55.5	48.3	48.3	51.2
No effect	8.1	9.3	18.6	2.5	3.3	10.1	10.2	5.1	13.7	7.9	7.0
Will make things worse	12.1	23.5	12.2	5.9	4.3	12.9	5.0	9.9	13.7	19.4	13.5
Don't know	30.3	23.6	24.6	52.5	34.5	23.3	36.3	28.8	24.3	24.4	27.6
No answer	0.4	0.1	0.9	0.0	0.0	0.0	0.0	0.0	0.0	0.0	0.8

Most of the research scientists, biotechnology companies promoting the research and the supermarket companies selling the foods recognise the potential risks which could be linked to novel foods developed through applications of modern biotechnology. They are also aware of consumer caution over accepting the novel foods. The scientists and the commercial companies understand the need to debate the ethical concerns and to develop a set of standards which regulate the development and use of DNA technology. The aims are to ensure an agreed responsible attitude to the work being undertaken, in relation to the wider environment, and to provide controls which can be implemented for the approval of individual products before they are released. Effective regulation should help to dispel public mistrust and win consumer confidence. Above all, people want to know that the food they eat is 'safe'. We must, however, remember that the 'public', or consumer, consists of diverse people, in different situations. They include old and young; Christians, Hindus and Muslims; rural and urban; from developed and from developing nations; scientists, politicians, farmers, economists, athletes and artists – people with a multitude of different social and cultural attitudes. They have diverse opinions, and inevitably hold different moral views on DNA technology.

Research with GMOs is done under controlled and confined conditions. In the development stages, genetically modified crops undergo extensive field trials before there is any question of releasing the GMO. The research tries to predict the possible influence of the GMO as well as assess any risk of harmful ecological or environmental change. Such trials are carried out in many locations, perhaps world-wide, and each transgenic crop is considered on an individual basis. Similar procedures are carried out for transgenic animals and microorganisms.

In the UK, all foods, before being released for public sale, have to meet a range of requirements, as laid down in the Food Safety Act, 1990. There are committees and regulatory bodies which look closely at novel foods and processes, including those involving genetically modified organisms. The Advisory Committee on Novel Foods and Processes is one such committee which has looked at a range of GM-derived foods, including tomato paste, herbicide-tolerant soya beans and chymosin from microbes. Members of this committee include research scientists, representatives from the food industry, consumer and environmental groups and medical experts. The network of steps required in Europe to market a novel food or food ingredient are summarised in Figure 4.19. A different series of steps is taken in the US to gain approval for novel foods or crops and this has led to some conflict in international trade. In considering GM foods, it is generally agreed in the UK that, in terms of safety, the food should be compared with an analogous conventional food to establish whether it is 'substantially equivalent'. It is also agreed that companies offering GM foods for sale should be encouraged to provide information about the product or ingredient which is readily accessible to the consumer. Such information can be supplied by means of the product label, or by information leaflets available at the time of purchase. Provided appropriate information is available and there is choice between GM and conventional food, it can then be an individual decision for each person to decide whether or not to consume GM food.

As the technology continues to develop, all individuals should be in a position to make an informed choice which is compatible with their own religious, cultural or personal beliefs. A biotechnology advisory working group (BAWG), comprising representatives from consumer organisations, agriculture, research, the major retailers and the food and related industries, has debated these issues at some length. The group has developed 'an extensive information framework, including Guidelines for communication and labelling of genetically modified foods'. In a statement made in 1997 BAWG supports a recommendation from the Food Advisory Committee, that food should 'be labelled if it contains a copy gene originally derived from: a human; an animal, the eating of which is restricted by some religions such as pigs for Muslims and cows for Hindus; or if it is a plant or microbial food and is modified with genes originally derived from any animal'. When implementing these guidelines, they need to be presented in a way that is easily understood by the consumer and be applied consistently to the full range of products as they become available. Foods containing or consisting of genetically modified organisms must be labelled. The information should let the consumer know if the composition or nutritional value is no longer equivalent to an existing food, whether there are any implications for health and whether any material in the food may give rise to ethical concerns.

It is perhaps not surprising that people have greeted modern biotechnology with cautious concern and this has probably played an important part in forcing public debate as it has with other biological issues. Nearly 150 years ago, public confidence was shaken by the suggestions put forward in Darwin's Theory of Evolution, yet today most people accept that there are close phylogenetic links between apes and humans. More recently people have been wary of accepting the reality of organ transplants and the possibilities of gene therapy. People continue to debate the issues surrounding birth control using the pill, abortion and *in vitro* fertilisation and here, as with modern biotechnology, we need to have access to information that enables us to understand the facts and the issues involved. We then need to keep a balanced perspective about DNA or gene technology and its role in society, now and in the 21st century. In 1929, the biologist J.B.S. Haldane had his eye on the future when he said, 'Why trouble to make compounds yourself when a bug will do it for you?'

For centuries people have eaten rice from plants infected with RSV (rice stripe virus). Do you think the same people would be happy to eat transgenic rice which contains the gene for the virus protein coat?

Do you think that herbicide resistant crop plants would encourage more spraying with herbicides or less use of herbicides?
What benefits might there be if the ability to fix nitrogen is transferred to cereal crops? Think about the economics, possibility of growing crops on marginal land, and environmental consequences in relation to use of fertilisers.

BIOTECHNOLOGY AND FOOD PRODUCTION

Compare the influence that biotechnology could have on crop production with the energy inputs of intensive farming methods. Make a case that biotechnology could help small-scale subsistence farmers in poor agricultural areas. Then list some of the worries that biotechnology would just increase profits for large multinational companies, in agriculture and in the food industry.

Modern farming practices, including monoculture and narrowing of the gene pool through selection of strains, tend to reduce biological diversity. How far do you think biotechnology can help *increase* biological diversity?

Do you think that all products which contain GMOs or GM-derived food should be labelled, or should the labelling be applied to all products which do not contain GM foods?
How, in practical terms, would a labelling directive be implemented? What information would you give on the label?

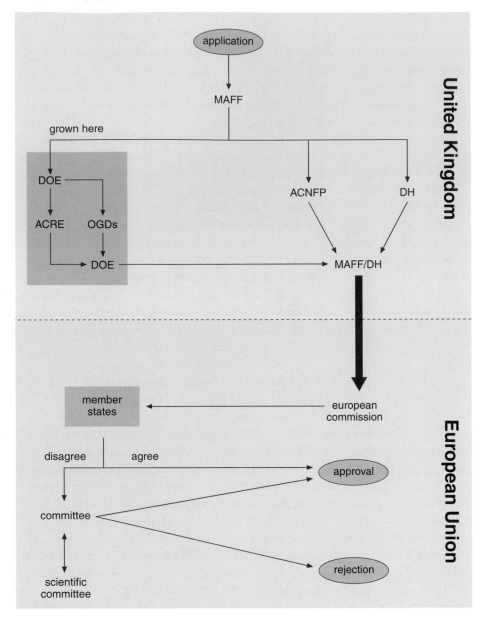

MAFF • Ministry of Agriculture, Fisheries and Food

DOE • Department of the Environment

DH • Department of Health

ACRW • Advisory Committee on Novel Foods and Processess

OGDs • Other government departments e.g. The Committee on the Toxicity of chemicals in food, consumer products and the environment (COT)), or the

Figure 4.19 Procedure (in 1997) for approval to market a novel food or food ingredients

Determination of calorific values of foods using a calorimeter

Introduction

A calorimeter, or heat of combustion apparatus, can be used to measure the calorific value of a sample of food. Combustion of the food in oxygen releases heat energy which will increase the temperature of the water contained in the apparatus. Measuring the rise in temperature of the water enables us to calculate the heat output of the food sample, and therefore the calorific value.

Materials

- Heat of combustion apparatus with nickel crucible
- Low voltage power supply
- Cylinder of oxygen fitted with reducing valve and regulator
- Thermometer
- Filter pump attached to tap
- Rubber tubing to connect oxygen and filter pump
- Measuring cylinder
- Electronic balance
- Suitable food sample, such as a small potato chip or toast, previously dried and kept in a desiccator

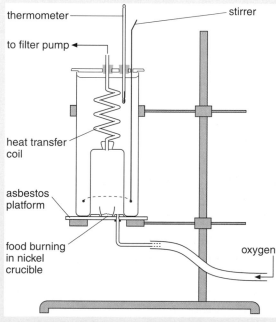

Figure P.1 A calorimeter used to determine the heat of combustion of food. An electric heating coil is used to ignite the food sample

Method

1 Fill the calorimeter jacket with water to cover the heat exchange coil, then tip the water into a measuring cylinder and record the volume. Return the water to the calorimeter.

2 Connect the apparatus to the oxygen supply, low voltage supply and filter pump, as shown in Figure P.1.

3 Weigh the nickel crucible and add a piece of suitable foodstuff.

4 Find and record the mass of food used.

5 Place the crucible centrally in the calorimeter and move the ignition coil so that it is just touching the food. Turn on the supply of oxygen and the filter pump.

6 Record the initial temperature of the water.

7 Ignite the food and then immediately move the ignition coil away from the crucible.

8 Move the stirrer steadily up and down including the doubled-walled area and the heat exchange coil. If necessary, adjust the flow rate of oxygen to keep the combustion steady.

9 Continue stirring for at least two minutes after the flame has gone out and record the maximum temperature reached by the water.

Results and discussion

1 Make a table to show the volume of water in the calorimeter, the mass of food used, the initial temperature and final temperature of the water, and the rise in temperature.

2 For comparative purposes, we can calculate the heat produced by the burning food by assuming that all the heat produced is transferred to the water. Naturally, this introduces an error, as it does not take into account the water equivalent of the apparatus itself. For more accurate determinations, the apparatus can be calibrated and a correction made.

3 If we assume that all the heat produced by the burning food is transferred to water and use the relationship that 1 calorie is the heat energy required to raise 1 g of water by 1 °C, then heat produced by food

PRACTICALS

(calories) = mass of water (g) × rise in temperature (°C)

4 Convert your result to joules, using the relationship: 1 calorie = 4.2 joules.

5 Compare your result with figures obtained from Food Tables. How closely does your result agree?

6 Consider the sources of error in this experiment.

Estimation of subcutaneous fat by skin-fold measurement

Introduction

A skinfold caliper is used to measure the thickness of a fold of skin with its underlying layer of subcutaneous fat. The calipers usually have a spring which exerts a standard pressure on the skin and an accurate scale to measure the thickness in millimetres. Measurements may be made from four sites, the back of the upper arm, front of upper arm, the back below the shoulder blade and on the side of the waist, or from just one site, such as the back of the upper arm. If four readings are taken, the sum of the readings, in mm, can be converted to percentage body fat using the tables given.

Materials

- Skin-fold caliper.
- Tables to convert readings to percentage body fat.

Method

1 If possible, take skinfold measurements from all four sites of a person. A faster, but less accurate estimation can be obtained using one site. If one site is to be used, this should be the back of the upper arm

2 Using Figures P.2 to P.5 to show where to take measurements, measure and record skinfold thickness from a volunteer.

3 Convert your readings to percentage body fat using Tables P.1, P.2, P.3 and P.4.

Results and discussion

1 Tabulate your results fully

2 What is the importance of measurement of body fat?

3 What is the ideal percentage body fat?

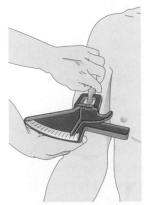

Figure P.2 Measuring skin-fold thickness at the front of the upper arm

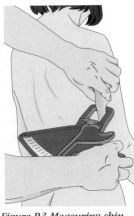

Figure P.3 Measuring skin-fold thickness at the back of the upper arm

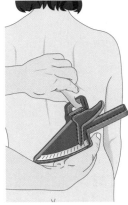

Figure P.4 Measuring skin-fold thickness on the back below shoulder blade

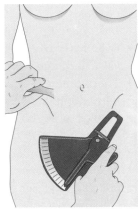

Figure P.5 Measuring skin-fold thickness on the side of waist

Quantitative estimation of sugars

Introduction

Concentrations of reducing sugars can be determined semi-quantitatively using Benedict's reagent and a range of colour standards. Quantitative estimations of glucose concentrations may be determined conveniently using suitable test strips, such as Diabur 5000. The concentration of sucrose can be estimated by first adding a drop of 10% invertase (sucrase) concentrate to 2 cm^3 of the solution to be tested and leaving for 30 minutes at room temperature. After enzyme treatment, the solution is tested for the presence of a reducing sugar. This method is preferable to acid hydrolysis.

Table P.1 *Percentage body fat for men using sum of measurements at all four locations*

Sum of skinfold measurements mm	Age 16–29	Age 30–49	Age 50+
20	8.1	12.1	12.5
22	9.2	13.2	13.9
24	10.2	14.2	15.1
26	11.2	15.2	16.3
28	12.1	16.1	17.4
30	12.9	16.9	18.5
35	14.7	18.7	20.8
40	16.3	20.3	22.8
45	17.7	21.8	24.7
50	19.0	23.0	26.3
55	20.2	24.2	27.8
60	21.2	25.3	29.1
65	22.2	26.3	30.4
70	23.2	27.2	31.5
75	24.0	28.0	32.6
80	24.8	28.8	33.7
85	25.6	29.6	34.6
90	26.3	30.3	35.5
95	27.0	31.0	36.5
100	27.6	31.7	37.3
110	28.8	32.9	38.8
120	29.9	34.0	40.2
130	31.0	35.0	41.5
140	31.9	36.0	42.8
150	32.8	36.8	43.9
160	33.6	37.7	45.0
170	34.4	38.5	46.0
180	35.2	39.2	47.0
190	35.9	39.9	47.9
200	36.5	40.6	48.8

Table P.2 *Percentage body fat for women using sum of measurements at all four locations*

Sum of skinfold measurements mm	Age 16–29	Age 30–49	Age 50+
14	9.4	14.1	17.0
16	11.2	15.7	18.6
18	12.7	17.1	20.1
20	14.1	18.4	21.4
22	15.4	19.5	22.6
24	16.5	20.6	23.7
26	17.6	21.5	24.8
28	18.6	22.4	25.7
30	19.5	23.3	26.6
35	21.6	25.2	28.6
40	23.4	26.8	30.3
45	25.0	28.3	31.9
50	26.5	29.6	33.2
55	27.8	30.8	34.6
60	29.1	31.9	35.7
65	30.2	32.9	36.7
70	31.2	33.9	37.7
75	32.2	34.7	38.6
80	33.1	35.6	39.5
85	34.0	36.3	40.4
90	34.8	37.1	41.1
95	35.6	37.8	41.9
100	36.3	38.5	42.6
110	37.7	39.7	43.9
120	39.0	40.8	45.1
130	40.2	41.9	46.2
140	41.3	42.9	47.3
150	42.3	43.8	48.2
160	43.2	44.7	49.1
170	44.6	45.5	50.0
180	45.0	46.2	50.8
190	45.8	46.9	51.6
200	46.6	47.6	52.3

Table P.3 *Percentage body fat for men using measurement on back of upper arm*

Skinfold thickness mm	Age 16–29	Age 30–49	Age 50+
3			12.1
4		14.4	15.7
5		16.6	18.6
6	10.8	18.6	20.6
7	12.5	20.2	22.9
8	13.9	21.5	24.6
9	15.2	22.6	26.2
10	16.4	23.6	27.6
11	17.4	24.5	28.8
12	18.4	25.3	30.0
13	19.3	26.1	31.1
14	20.1	26.8	32.1
15	20.9	27.5	33.0
16	21.6	28.1	33.9
17	22.3	28.7	34.7
18	22.9	29.2	35.5
19	23.5	29.8	36.2
20	24.1	30.3	36.9
22	25.2	31.2	38.2
24	26.2	32.1	39.5
26	27.1	32.9	40.6
28	28.0	33.6	41.6
30	28.8	34.3	42.6
32	29.5	34.9	43.5
34	30.3	35.5	44.3
36	30.9	36.1	45.2
38	31.6	36.7	45.9
40	32.2	37.2	46.7
45	33.6	38.4	48.4
50	34.8	39.4	49.9
55	35.9	40.4	51.3
60	37.0	41.3	52.5
65	37.9	42.1	53.7
70	38.8	42.9	54.8
75	39.7	43.6	55.8
80	40.5	44.3	56.8

Table P.4 *Percentage body fat for women using measurement on back of upper arm*

Skinfold thickness mm	Age 16–29	Age 30–49	Age 50+
4		11.2	12.6
5	10.8	14.0	15.8
6	13.3	16.4	18.4
7	15.3	18.5	20.7
8	17.2	20.2	22.7
9	18.8	21.8	24.5
10	20.2	23.2	26.1
11	21.5	24.5	27.5
12	22.8	25.7	28.8
13	23.9	26.8	30.1
14	24.9	27.8	31.2
15	25.9	28.8	32.3
16	26.8	29.7	33.3
17	27.7	30.5	34.2
18	28.5	31.3	35.1
19	29.3	32.1	36.0
20	30.0	32.8	36.8
22	31.4	34.1	38.3
24	32.6	35.4	39.7
26	33.8	36.5	41.0
28	34.9	37.9	42.2
30	35.9	38.6	43.3
32	36.9	39.5	44.4
34	37.8	40.4	45.3
36	38.6	41.2	46.3
38	39.4	42.0	47.2
40	40.2	42.8	48.0
45	42.0	44.5	50.0
50	43.6	46.1	51.8
55	45.0	47.5	53.4
60	46.3	48.8	54.8
65	47.6	50.0	56.2
70	48.7	51.1	57.5
75	49.8	52.2	58.7
80	50.8	53.1	59.8

PRACTICALS

Materials

- Range of food samples to be tested
- Mortar and pestle
- Beaker to use as boiling water bath
- Test tubes
- Diabur 5000 reagent strips
- Benedict's reagent
- Pipettes or syringes
- 10% invertase (sucrase) concentrate
- Standard glucose solutions: 2.0, 1.0, 0.5, 0.1, 0.05, 0.02 and 0.01 per cent.

WEAR EYE PROTECTION

Method

1 To produce a range of colour standards, use a series of glucose solutions of known concentration. Add 0.3 cm³ of each of these solutions to a series of appropriately labelled test tubes, each containing 5.0 cm³ of Benedict's reagent. These test tubes should then be placed in a boiling water bath for 8 minutes, then left to cool in air.

2 To estimate the concentration of reducing sugars in the food samples, pipette 5.0 cm³ of Benedict's reagent into a test tube and add 0.3 cm³ of the solution to be tested. Heat in a boiling water bath for 8 minutes, leave to cool, then compare the colour produced with the colour standards.

3 If using Diabur test strips, a strip should be dipped into the solution to be tested, removed, and the colours produced compared with the colour chart after two minutes. This method is specific for glucose, and will give quantitative results.

Results and discussion

1 Tabulate all your results suitably.
2 Present the results in a suitable graphical form.
3 What are the sources of error in this experiment? How could it be improved?

Further work

1 Estimate the reducing sugar content of a range of fruit juices, both fresh and packaged.
2 Investigate the changes in reducing sugar content during, for example, the ripening of fruit.
3 Find out about other quantitative methods for the determination of reducing sugar content.

Quantitative estimation of ascorbic acid

Introduction

Ascorbic acid (vitamin C) is a reducing agent and can be detected using a dye, DCPIP (phenol-indo-2:6-dichlorophenol). DCPIP is blue in the oxidised form (which will turn red in acidic solutions) and turns pale yellowish-brown when reduced. During the test, the tubes should not be shaken as atmospheric oxygen can re-oxidise the DCPIP, giving inaccurate results.

Materials

- 0.1% ascorbic acid solution (1 mg ascorbic acid per cm³)
- 0.1% aqueous DCPIP solution. This should be made up fresh each time
- Samples of fruit juice, such as lemon, grapefruit, lime, grape and apple
- Test tubes
- 1 cm³ syringes fitted with needles.

Safety note: take care when handling syringes fitted with needles

Method

1 Use a syringe or pipette to transfer exactly 1.0 cm³ of DCPIP solution into a test tube.

2 Fill another 1 cm³ syringe with the standard 0.1% ascorbic acid solution and, keeping the end of the needle below the surface of the DCPIP, carefully add the ascorbic acid solution until the DCPIP is decolourised. Do not shake the mixture, it may be gently stirred using the needle.

3 Record the volume of ascorbic acid solution required to decolourise the DCPIP.

4 Repeat this test with 1.0 cm³ of fresh DCPIP solution and fruit juice, such as lemon juice.

5 Record the volume of fruit juice required to decolourise the DCPIP.

6 Repeat the procedure with samples of different fruit juices.

Results and discussion

1 Record your results in a table.
2 Calculate the concentration of ascorbic acid in the fruit juice sample, using the following relationship. Suppose that the volume of standard ascorbic acid solution required to decolourise 1.0 cm³ of DCPIP

was x cm³, and the volume of fruit juice required to decolourise the same volume of DCPIP solution was y cm³, then the concentration of ascorbic acid in the fruit juice sample will be $x \div y$ mg of ascorbic acid per cm³.

3 Present your results in a suitable graphical form so that the ascorbic acid content of the different fruits can be compared.

Further work

1 Investigate differences in the ascorbic acid content between fresh and bottled fruit juice, or juice from a carton.

2 Investigate changes in the ascorbic acid content of fruit during storage.

3 Investigate the effect of boiling on ascorbic acid content of fruit juice.

Enzymic browning in fruit and vegetables

Introduction

Damage to fruit and vegetables, such as cutting or bruising, results in changes to their metabolism. One of the most obvious changes is browning of damaged tissues, which results in both an undesirable colour change and spoilage of the texture. This dicolouration can result from handling, processing, or packaging of fruit and vegetables, and is referred to as adventitious browning.

Adventitious browning is due to the action of enzymes on a variety of substrates, resulting in the production of, for example, quinone which polymerises to form coloured compounds. This reaction occurs when cells are damaged and exposed to oxygen. The enzymes responsible for browning are referred to by different names, such as phenolase, polyphenolase and polyphenol oxidase. These are a group of different enzymes, including tyrosinase and catecholase. Like all enzymes, they are sensitive to changes in temperature and pH, and can be inactivated by the presence of certain ions, such as heavy metals.

Materials

- Suitable fruits and vegetables, such as apples (Bramleys are recommended), peaches, apricots, bananas, pears or potatoes

- Kitchen knives - take care when handling these
- Mortars and pestles
- Citric acid – disodium hydrogen orthophosphate buffer solutions, pH range from 2.0 to 8.0
- Test tubes or boiling tubes
- Beakers or water baths
- Thermometers

Method

1 An initial experiment should be carried out to investigate the time taken for the tissue to brown when cut, broken, or pulped using a mortar and pestle.

2 Investigate the effect of pH on the rate of browning, by immersing* suitable pieces of tissue in buffer solutions.

3 Investigate the effect of temperature on the rate of browning, using water baths at a range of temperatures from 20 °C to 80 °C.

*Browning will be slow if the pieces are immersed in solution.

Results and discussion

1 Tabulate your results fully, showing the effects of different factors on the rate of browning.

2 Plot graphs to show the effects of changes in pH and temperature on the rate of browning.

3 Describe and explain the effects of the different treatments on enzymic browning.

4 What are the sources of error in this experiment?

5 Discuss the importance of your results in relation to handling, packaging and processing of food and vegetables.

Further work

1 Investigate the effects of other factors on browning, such as freezing, the use of preservatives, including salt, sugar and sulphur dioxide. Campden tablets can be used as a source of sulphur dioxide.

2 Investigate the effects of copper ions on the activity of phenolases, using copper sulphate solution.

3 Compare the rates of browning of different varieties of the same fruit.

PRACTICALS

Identification of food constituents in milk

Introduction

The purpose of this practical is to identify and, where possible, quantify the food constituents of milk. There are a number of possibilities for comparing the content of different types of milk, and of milk treated in different ways, such as pasteurised, sterilised and UHT.

Materials

- Samples of different types of milk
- Benedict's reagent
- Biuret reagent (Dissolve 8 g of sodium hydroxide in 800 cm³ of distilled water. Add 45 g of sodium potassium tartrate and dissolve. Then add 5 g of copper sulphate; dissolve, and add 5 g of potassium iodide. Finally make up to 1.0 dm³ with distilled water. Each reagent must be fully dissolved before adding the next. The solution should be kept in a dark bottle.
- Sudan III in ethanolic solution
- Beaker to use as boiling water bath
- Pipettes or syringes
- Test tubes
- Microscope slides and coverslips
- Microscope

IRRITANT
Sodium hydroxide

HIGHLY FLAMMABLE
sudan III in ethanolic solution

Method

1. Estimate the reducing sugar content of the milk samples, using the method described in Practical: Quantitative estimation of sugars (page 84).
2. To test for proteins, place 2 cm³ of the sample to be tested in a test tube and add an equal volume of biuret reagent. A purple-violet colour develops slowly, the intensity of which is proportional to the protein content.
3. To show the presence of fat, add a minute drop of Sudan III solution to a drop of milk on a microscope slide and apply a cover slip. Examine using a microscope; an emulsion of fat droplets should be visible.

Results and discussion

1. Prepare a table to record your observations using each test.
2. Compare the reducing sugar content, protein and fat content of each sample of milk.

Further work

The relative density of milk samples can be compared by determining the time taken for a drop of milk to fall through a solution of copper(II) sulphate. A layer of copper proteinate forms around the drop, which prevents the milk dispersing. Use a 100 cm³ measuring cylinder, filled approximately 5 cm above the 100 cm³ mark with 0.1 mol dm⁻³ copper(II) sulphate solution. Introduce one drop of milk, using a syringe fitted with a needle, just below the surface of the copper(II) sulphate solution and record the time taken for the drop to fall between the 100 cm³ and 10 cm³ marks. Repeat using different types of milk.

The resazurin test, methylene blue test and turbidity test

Introduction

The tests in this practical investigate the freshness of milk, by using methods which indicate the activity of bacteria, and also the effectiveness of pasteurisation and sterilisation.

Resazurin is an indicator which shows metabolic activity of bacteria. The indicator is blue in the oxidised state but changes, when reduced, through pink to white. Although this test does not show the types of bacteria present, it can be used as a means of comparing the bacterial content of milk samples. Tubes containing milk which change colour to white, pink or white mottling have failed the test.

Methylene blue is a sensitive redox indicator which, like resazurin, shows bacterial activity in the milk sample. Methylene blue is decolourised when reduced, so recording the time taken for the blue colour to disappear gives an indication of bacterial activity in the milk sample.

The turbidity test is used to check for the efficiency of sterilisation. The procedure depends on changes in the properties of milk proteins after treatment at different temperatures and after the addition of ammonium sulphate. After addition of ammonium sulphate and filtration, the filtrate should remain clear on boiling if the sterilisation procedure has been effective.

(a) The resazurin test

Materials

- Milk samples
- Resazurin tablets
- Distilled water
- Pipettes or syringes
- Sterile screw-capped containers, such as universal bottles
- Water bath at 37 °C.

Method

1 Dissolve one resazurin tablet in 50 cm^3 of distilled water.
2 Add 1.0 cm^3 of this solution to 10.0 cm^3 of milk to be tested in a sterile container. Replace the lid, label the container and invert once to mix the contents.
3 Incubate in a water bath at 37 °C, filled so that the level of water is just over the level of milk in the container.
4 Set up a control tube containing 10.0 cm^3 of boiled milk plus 1.0 cm^3 resazurin solution.
5 Examine the samples after 10 minutes and note any colour changes.
6 Replace in the water bath and examine again after 1 hour.
7 Compare the colour of each sample with that of the control tube, which should remain blue.

(b) The methylene blue test

Materials

- Milk samples
- 5.0% acetaldehyde (ethanal) solution. Add a few drops of phenolphthalein indicator, followed by a dilute solution of sodium carbonate until the mixture just turns pink.
- 0.01% methylene blue solution.
- Distilled water
- Pipettes or syringes
- Test tubes
- Aluminium foil
- Water bath at 40 °C.

Method

1 Measure 5.0 cm^3 of pasteurised milk into a test tube, add 1.0 cm^3 of the acetaldehyde solution and 1.0 cm^3 of methylene blue. Mix the contents by shaking the tube gently, then cover the top of the tube with a small piece of aluminium foil.
2 Stand the tube in a water bath at 40 °C and note the time taken for the methylene blue to become decolourised. A blue ring may remain at the top of the sample.
3 Repeat this procedure with other samples of milk.

(c) The turbidity test

Materials

- Milk samples: sterilised, pasteurised, pasteurised and boiled for 5 minutes
- Ammonium sulphate
- Electronic balance
- Conical flasks, 50 cm^3
- Measuring cylinder, 100 cm^3
- Filter funnels and filter paper
- Test tubes
- Beaker to use as a boiling water bath
- Pipettes or syringes
- Bench lamp.

Method

1 Weigh 4 g of ammonium sulphate and transfer to a conical flask.
2 Add 20 cm^3 of the milk sample to be tested to the ammonium sulphate.
3 Shake the flask for at least 1 minute to dissolve the ammonium sulphate.
4 Leave the flask to stand for 5 minutes.
5 Filter the contents of the flask and transfer 5.0 cm^3 of the filtrate to a test tube.
6 Place the test tube in a boiling water bath and leave for 5 minutes.
7 Cool the tube in a beaker of cold water, then examine the contents by holding the tube in front of a bench lamp.

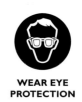

WEAR EYE PROTECTION

Results and discussion

1 Record all your results in a suitable table.
2 Compare the results of each test for the different samples of milk used and comment on their significance.
3 Find out about the possible health risks associated with untreated (raw) milk. What steps are taken to minimise these risks?

PRACTICALS

Investigating weight loss in packaged foods

Introduction

Various different packaging materials, such as paper, PVC films and cling wrap, are used for fruit and vegetables. These can help to reduce water loss, and also modify the atmosphere surrounding the produce and thereby increase the shelf-life. If fruits are enclosed in a plastic film, they continue to respire, using up oxygen and producing carbon dioxide and water. The increase in carbon dioxide reduces the metabolic rate of many fruits and increases their shelf-life. However, if a covering film is impermeable to water vapour, the increase in humidity surrounding the produce encourages the growth of fungal or bacterial spores, resulting in food spoilage.

The purpose of this practical is to investigate the effect of different packaging materials on weight loss, and changes in the appearance of fruit and vegetables.

Materials

- Containers, such as small plastic boxes or punnets
- Packaging materials such as thin PVC film, cling wrap, paper
- Selection of fruit and vegetables; apples, mushrooms, small lettuces and carrots are suitable
- Electronic balance

Method

1 Weigh the containers and packaging materials separately, introduce the produce, wrap suitably and weigh again. Record the mass of produce. Remember to include one uncovered container as a control.
2 Re-weigh at suitable intervals. This will depend on the nature of the produce, it may be necessary to carry out a preliminary experiment. Record the mass of each container of produce.
3 If you have access to a refrigerator, place one set of containers in the salad compartment and leave one set at room temperature. Record mass as before.

4 Record changes in the appearance of the produce.

Results and discussion

1 Record all your results in a suitable table.
2 Calculate the percentage change in mass of the produce.
3 Plot graphs to show percentage change in mass against time.
4 Compare the results for each type of packaging material.
5 What effect did temperature have on the rate of loss in mass?
6 Consider which factors are important in the choice of packaging materials.

Further work

This experiment lends itself to a number of investigations into ways of increasing the shelf-life of fruit and vegetables, by slowing deterioration. It is possible to modify the composition of the atmosphere in the container by, for example, including a small beaker of soda water to increase the concentration of carbon dioxide. Alternatively, you could try including a small amount of potassium permanganate, which will remove ethene (ethylene) from the atmosphere in the container. Remember to include suitable controls in your experiments.

1 Investigate the effect of raising the concentration of carbon dioxide on the shelf-life of lettuce.
2 Investigate the effect of removing ethene (ethylene) from the atmosphere on the keeping qualities of bananas.

Changes in food during the process of fermentation

Introduction

In Chapter 4, we have described some of the chemical changes which occur in foods during the process of fermentation. In this practical, we look at the changes in pH which occur in milk during the formation of yoghurt. Bacteria in the starter culture ferment milk sugars to produce organic acids, such as methanoic and lactic acid, and consequently the pH will fall.

Materials

- UHT milk
- Natural yoghurt to use as a starter culture
- Boiling tubes
- Pipettes or syringes
- Cling film
- Glass stirring rod
- pH meter (if unavailable, narrow range pH papers could be used as an alternative)
- Water bath at 43 °C.

Method

1 Transfer 10.0 cm^3 of UHT into a boiling tube then add 1.0 cm^3 of natural yoghurt.
2 Record the pH of the mixture, cover the tube with cling film, and incubate in a water bath at 43 °C.
3 Record the pH and changes in the appearance of the yoghurt at intervals of 30 minutes for up to 5 hours.
4 Dispose of incubated milk carefully after completing the practical. Equipment should be sterilised after use.

Results and discussion

1 Record your results in a table, then plot a graph to show changes in the pH during fermentation.
2 Describe the changes which occurred in pH and in the appearance of the yoghurt during fermentation.
3 Prepare a flow chart to show the stages in industrial yoghurt manufacture.

Further work

1 Investigate the changes in pH during production of yoghurt using different types of milk, such as cow's, ewe's or goat's.
2 Investigate changes in pH during production of yoghurt using lactose-reduced milk, such as Lactolite, or starter cultures containing *Lactobacillus acidophilus* and *Bifidobacterium bifidum*.
3 Devise a method to investigate changes in reducing sugar content during the production of yoghurt.
4 The principle of this experiment could be extended to, for example, measurement of changes in pH during fermentation of cabbage to make sauerkraut.

Perception of sweetness in drinks or food

Introduction

The degree of sweetness of sugars varies, and some sugars therefore will taste sweeter than others. Sucrose is used as the standard reference substance for sweetness and the degrees of sweetness of other sugars are usually compared with that of sucrose. The aim of this practical is to compare the taste of different sugars and to arrange them in order of apparent sweetness. *Safety note*: If this activity is to take place in the laboratory ensure that lab benches have been thoroughly cleaned, and that sugars are not contaminated. The sugars should not be stored with other chemicals.

Materials

- Disposable plastic cups
- Supply of drinking water
- 4 per cent solutions of sucrose, lactose, maltose, glucose and fructose, made up in drinking water. Label the solutions A, B, C, etc.

Method

1 Taste each of the solutions in turn, rinsing your mouth out with water between each solution. Decide which solution tastes (a) the most sweet (b) the least sweet.
2 Arrange the solutions in order of sweetness, from the most sweet to the least.

Results and discussion

1 Record your results in a suitable table, including the identity of each solution.
2 Refer to Table 2.5 on page 25. To what extent do your results agree with these values for relative sweetness? Suggest reasons for any differences.

Further work

1 Investigate the threshold concentrations, by tasting a range of concentrations of each sugar, for example, 0.001, 0.01, 0.05, 0.1 and 0.2 mol per dm^3.
2 Compare the relative sweetness and note any 'aftertaste' of artificial sweeteners such as aspartame and saccharin.
3 Consider how you might develop this practical to include statistical treatment of the results.

Examination questions

Chapter 1

1 The table below refers to constituents of diet and the effects of deficiencies in the supply of these constituents. Complete the table by writing the appropriate word or words in the empty boxes

Constituent of the diet	Effect of deficiency
Retinol	
	Bleeding from small blood vessels and gums
Essential amino acids	
Fibre	
	Anaemia

(Total 5 marks)

2 Read through the following passage about enzymes and their industrial uses, then write on the dotted lines the most appropriate word or words to complete the account.

As much as 75% of the world's adult population may be unable to tolerate and digest the sugar in milk, and so this sugar is removed during the manufacture of some milk products. This is done using the enzyme .... which hydrolyses the milk sugar into .... and .... Unlike the sugar in milk, these are both .... sugars. They are both .... than milk sugar, so milk products treated in this way are particularly useful in the manufacture of confectionery.

(Total 5 marks)

3 In formulating a diet, it is necessary to consider the nutritional value of different component foods.

The *biological value* (BV) of a source of protein is defined as the percentage of absorbed protein that is converted into body protein.

The *digestibility* of a source of protein is a measure of the proportion of that protein which is broken down into amino acids during digestion.

The *net protein utilisation* (NPU) is the percentage of protein eaten that is retained by the body.

The relationship between the BV, digestibility and NPU is given by the following equation.

$$NPU = BV \times digestibility$$

The BV and NPU values of six different sources of protein are shown in the table below.

Source of protein	BV value	NPU value
Egg	98	96
Meat	80	76
Milk	77	71
Soya flour	70	60
Maize	36	31
Gelatin	0	0

(a) (i) Calculate the digestibility of egg protein. Show your working. (2 marks)

(ii) The digestibility of soya flour protein is 0.86. Comment on the difference between this figure for soya flour and that calculated for egg protein in (a) (i).

(b) The BV of a protein depends on the content of essential amino acids.

(i) Explain what is meant by the term *essential amino acid*. (2 marks)

(ii) Suggest why gelatin has a BV of 0. (1 mark)

(iii) Suggest why, in the foods given in the table, most animal proteins have a higher BV than the plant proteins. (2 marks)

(c) Suggest a reason why protein malnutrition is common in countries where cassava (manioc) is staple diet. (2 marks)

(Total 12 marks)

4 Body mass index (BMI) is used as a measure of obesity which can be an indicator of long term health

A number of people agreed to have their mass and height measured to determine their BMI.

The results are shown in the table below.

Person	Mass / kg	Height / m	BMI
A	59.67	1.75	19.48
B	65.03	1.70	22.50
C	63.92	1.65	23.48
D	66.56	1.60	26.00
E	58.80	1.55	

Body mass index (BMI) is given by the equation

$$\text{BMI} = \frac{\text{mass} / \text{kg}}{(\text{height} / \text{m})^2}$$

For healthy people, BMI should lie in the range of 20 to 25. A BMI outside this range is regarded as a potential health risk.

(a) (i) Calculate the BMI for person E. Show your working.   (2 marks)

   (ii) State which of the people would be considered as overweight.   (1 mark)

   (iii) Suggest *three* possible long-term harmful effects of having a high BMI.   (3 marks)

(b)   Suggest *two* factors which should be taken into account when interpreting BMI values.   (2 marks)

(c)   Explain the relationship between physical activity and body mass.   (3 marks)
                                (Total 11 marks)

Chapter 2

1 Explain what is meant by each of the following terms.
   (a)   Antioxidants   (2 marks)

   (b)   E numbers   (2 marks)

(c)   Flavour enhancers   (2 marks)
                                (Total 6 marks)

2 It is suggested that fibre in the diet has an influence on the occurrence of cancer of the colon and diverticular disease.

The graph below shows the mortality from cancer of the colon for nine different areas of Britain plotted against the intake of fibre in the diet.

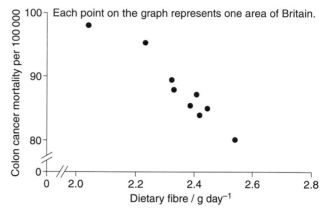

(a) (i) Comment on the relationships between fibre in the diet and mortality from cancer of the colon.   (3 marks)

   (ii) Explain why increasing the intake of dietary fibre may affect the incidence of cancer of the colon.   (2 marks)

(b)   In a study of diverticular disease in Oxford the following results were recorded.

   A Over half the population over 70 years of age had diverticular disease

   B The occurrence of diverticular disease was much lower in vegetarians.

   C There was no significant difference in the occurrence of diverticular disease in males and females.

Suggest a reason for each of these findings
                                (3 marks)

(c)   Suggest *three* other effects on nutrition that arise as a result of a diet high in fibre and low in animal protein.   (3 marks)
                                (Total 11 marks)

EXAMINATION QUESTIONS

Chapter 3

1   Many types of fruit and vegetables are pre-packed to increase the time they will stay fresh when stored.

(a)   State *two* metabolic processes that occur in stored fruit.   (2 marks)

(b)   The diagram below shows a package containing fresh apples.

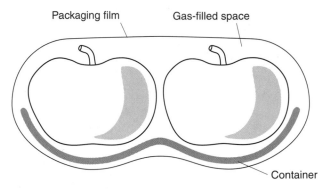

Packaging film   Gas-filled space

Container

Select *two* features of the packaging shown in the diagram and explain how each of them helps to prolong the storage time of the apples.   (4 marks)

(Total 6 marks)

2   Give an account of chemical and biological which occur in foods during storage.

(Total 10 marks)

Chapter 4

1   Single cell protein can be produced by growing the bacterium *Methylophilus methylotrophus* in a fermenter. The industrial process is outlined in the diagram below. Single cell protein is used as a supplement to animal feed.

(a) (i) State two roles for the methanol used in the process.   (2 marks)

(ii) State the role of the ammonia used in the process.   (1 mark)

(b)   Suggest why the fermenter is kept at 40 °C.   (1 mark)

(c)   Explain why single cell protein produced from bacterial cells used as an animal feed supplement rather than as human food.   (2 marks)

(Total 6 marks)

2   Give an account of the use of microorganisms to modify foods by fermentation

(Total 10 marks)

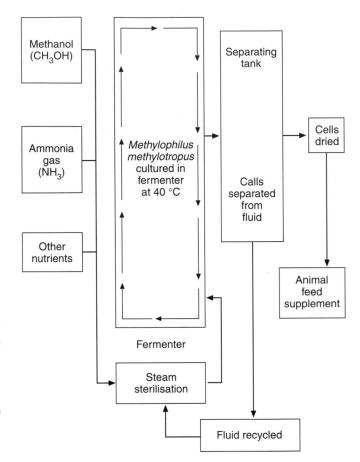

Methanol
(CH_3OH)

Ammonia
gas
(NH_3)

Other
nutrients

*Methylophilus
methylotropus*
cultured in
fermenter
at 40 °C

Separating
tank

Cells
dried

Calls
separated
from
fluid

Animal
feed
supplement

Fermenter

Steam
sterilisation

Fluid recycled

EDEXCEL Foundation, London Examinations accepts no responsibility whatsoever for the accuracy or method of working in the answers given.

In the mark schemes, the following symbols are used:

; indicates separate marking points
/ indicates alternative marking points
eq means correct equivalent points are accepted

Chapter 1

1

Constituent of the diet	Effect of deficiency
Retinol	mucous membrane degeneration / night blindness / xerophthalmia / complete blindness in children;
ascorbic acid / vitamin C ;	Bleeding from small blood vessels and gums
Essential amino acids	failure of protein production / failure of growth / eq. ;
Fibre	constipation / cancer of colon / diverticular disease / eq. ;
iron / Fe ;	Anaemia

2   As much as 75% of the world's adult population may be unable to tolerate and digest the sugar in milk, and so this sugar is removed during the manufacture of some milk products. This is done using the enzyme *lactase / β–galactosidase*; which hydrolyses the milk sugar into *glucose*; and *galactose*;. Unlike the sugar in milk, these are both *monosaccharide*; sugars. They are both *sweeter / more soluble*; than milk sugar, so milk products treated in this way are particularly useful in the manufacture of confectionery.

(Total 5 marks)

3   *(a)* (i)   96/98; 0.979 / 0.98 ;   (2 marks)

    (ii) egg more digestible / soya flour less digestible ; correct use of figures / difference 0.12; soya flour of plant origin; some trapped in cells; by insoluble cellulose; cells not digested / protein not exposed to digestive enzymes;   (3 marks)

(b) (i)   needed for production of human proteins; cannot be produced by the body; must be obtained from the diet;   (2 marks)

    (ii) absence of essential amino acids / no tryptophan / none retained by body / none absorbed ;

    (iii) contain all / most of the essential amino acids / OR converse for plants ; in the right proportions;   (2 marks)

(c)   cassava low in protein / not all protein retained / absorbed ; cassava low in essential amino acids; some completely missing ; supply of dietary protein dependent on other foods ; little / no animal protein in diet / eq. ;   (2 marks)
(Total 12 marks)

4   *(a)* (i)   58.80 ÷ (1.55)^2 ; 24.47 / 24.5 ;   (2 marks)

    (ii) person D ;   (1 mark)

    (iii) coronary heart disease / atherosclerosis / high blood pressure / hypertension / stroke / angina ;
increased danger of developing diabetes ;
increased likelihood of pulmonary problems / breathlessness ;
damage to joints by carrying excess weight / eq.; gall bladder disease ;
skin infection from skin folds ;
increased surgical risk eq. ;   (3 marks)

(b)   gender ; age ; general state of health ; lifestyle / level of physical activity ; pregnancy ;   (2 marks)

(c)   any change in level of physical activity may affect body mass ; increased physical activity increases energy expenditure / converse ; more exercise and no increased energy intake reduces body mass / eq. ; increased exercise increases muscle bulk ; this may increase body mass.   (3 marks)
(Total 11 marks)

MARK SCHEMES

Chapter 2

1 *(a)* prevent rancidity in fatty / lipid-rich foods / eq. ; maintain freshness / prevent browning in fruit; by combining with free radicals / remove free radicals from body ; e.g. vitamin C / vitamin E / eq. ; (2 marks)

(b) catalogue / list of a range of chemicals added to food / additives ; approved for use in EEC / eq. ; natural and artificial food additives ; any ref. to being named on labels / legal requirement / eq. ; (2 marks)

(c) substances added to food to improve taste / flavour ; or to bring out the natural flavour / not in themselves flavours ; e.g. monosodium glutamate / MSG / salt / eq. ; (2 marks)
(Total 10 marks)

2 *(a)* (i) mortality falls as dietary intake increases ; areas with similar dietary intake have similar mortalities ; sensible use of figures ; small increase in fibre has large effect ; (3 marks)

(ii) increases bulk of stools ; raises speed of passage through intestine; carcinogens move through gut more quickly ; fibre adsorbs carcinogens ; (2 marks)

(b) A weakening of the gut wall with age / thickening of gut wall with age / lower dietary fibre in diet / poor diet when young ;

B higher fibre intake / higher vegetable / cereal intake *or* cereals, vegetables contain a lot of fibre ;

C no hormonal difference / no dietary difference / no genetic difference / not sex-linked ; (3 marks)

(c) poor absorption / lack / eq. of iron ; reduced uptake / lack / eq. of calcium ; shortage of / lack of essential amino acids / or ref. to kwashiorkor ; (2 marks)
(Total 10 marks)

3 shortage of fat / fatty acids / fat soluble vitamins ; (3 marks)
(Total 11 marks)

Chapter 3

1 *(a)* *Any two from*: ripening / colour change ; breakdown of cell wall / pectinase activity ; respiration / oxidation / glycolysis / Krebs cycle ; breakdown / hydrolysis / conversion of starch to sugars ; autolysis / reduction with vitamin C ; (2 marks)

(b) *container* : rigid / tough / eq. / holds apples in place ; to protect from mechanical / physical damage / or bruising ;
film : if partially permeable; to allow escape of water vapour / gas exchange / prevention of increase in gas pressure / reduce fungal growth / keeps out microorganisms / prevents anaerobic respiration ;
if permeable ; keeps out microorganisms / prevents water loss / water gain ;
gas : if carbon dioxide / nitrogen / inert gases ; prevents aerobic respiration / oxidation / slows ripening / prevents physical damage ;
if air ; allows aerobic respiration / prevents physical damage ;
if MA ; comment about ripening / prevents physical damage ; (4 marks)
(Total 10 marks)

2 enzymic action on organic substances ; loss of protein ; textural changes / softening / ref. to frost damage ; (produced by) autolysis ; comment on meat becoming more tender ; (enzymic) browning of fruit / apples ; loss of vitamins ; 7 particularly vitamin C ; oxidation of fats / ref. to free radicals ; comment on rancidity ; respiration uses up sugars ; lowered pH / pH change ; spoilage by microorganisms / named e.g. mould growth ; production of toxins e.g. botulism / *Staphylococcus aureus* ; *(a)* bacterial action produces new substances ; example such as lactic acid / organic acids / may produce 'off' flavours / reduce palatability / ethanol ; colour change ; *(a)* loss of water; *(b)* loss of CO_2 ; shrivelling of fresh food / named e.g.; *(a)* ripening / ref. to ethene; *(b)* colour change / flavour change ; conversion of starch to sugar ; sprouting in stored vegetables / e.g. ;
(Total 10 marks)

Chapter 4

1 (a) (i) carbon source ;
          energy source / respiratory substrate ;
                                    (2 marks)

      (ii) nitrogen source / eq. for production of
           protein / amino acid ;   (1 mark)

   (b)   optimum / ideal temperature for bacterial
            growth ;   (1 mark)

   (c)   high nucleic acid content ; causes health
            problems in humans / causes gout ;
            expensive to remove nucleic acids / too
            expensive to produce for humans ;
            inadequate essetial amino acids ; not
            palatable / eq. / bland / needs to be
            flavoured ;   (2 marks)
                                    (Total 6 marks)

2   reference to the anaerobic respiration of yeast
    producing alcohol and carbon dioxide ; explanation
    of roles of enzymes in hydrolysis of carbohydrate
    substrates ; role of yeast in bread making causing
    fermentation of dough ; role of proteolytic enzymes
    in yeast on flour proteins ; comment on result of
    processes in terms of final product, e.g. light spongy
    texture ; role of yeast in conversion of grape juice /
    eq. to wine ; credit for specific detail of process ;
    conversion of alcohol in beer / cider / wine to
    vinegar; by *Acetobacter* ; aerobic fermentation /
    oxygen required ; ethanol to ethanoic acid ; souring
    of milk by lactose-fermenting / lactic acid bacteria in
    initial stages of cheese manufacture ; credit
    reference to named bacteria / *Streptococcus* spp. ;
    ferment sugars / lactose to lactic acid ; pH falls ;
    reference to the action of bacteria in the ripening of
    cheese ; role of lactic acid bacteria in the production
    of yoghurt from milk ; use of *Lactobacillus
    bulgaricus* and *Streptococcus thermophilus* in
    starter culture ; replication of the streptococci
    producing compounds giving flavour / creamy
    texture ; as pH falls, lactobacilli replicate producing
    lactic acid and ethanal ; soya milk (from soya beans)
    fermented to form tofu ; soy sauce production by
    fermentation with *Aspergillus / Candida* / eq. ;
    sauerkraut produced by fermentation of sugars in
    cabbage by lactic acid bacteria ; credit for correct,
    qualified references to other fermentation processes
    in the modification of foods as appropriate ;
                                    (Total 10 marks)

Index